"Dr. Agatston is a noted cardiologist who's made many contributions, but *The South Beach Diet* may be his best. Importantly, this is not 'another diet book.' This is a book about health and well-being. Dr. Agatston does an outstanding job of explaining the importance of the types of food we eat and its impact on preventing illnesses, such as coronary heart disease and diabetes. Not only will you feel better if you follow his diet, but you will look and live better."

—Randolph P. Martin, M.D., director of noninvasive cardiology at Emory University Hospital, Atlanta

---

For years, cardiologist Arthur Agatston, M.D., urged his patients to lose weight for the sake of their hearts, but every diet was too hard to follow or its restrictions were too harsh. Some were downright dangerous. Nobody seemed to be able to stick with low-fat regimens for any length of time. And a diet is useless if you can't stick with it.

So Dr. Agatston developed his own. *The South Beach Diet* isn't complicated, and it doesn't require that you go hungry. You'll enjoy normal-size helpings of meat, poultry, and fish. You'll also eat eggs, low-fat cheese, nuts, and vegetables. Snacks are required. You'll learn to avoid the bad carbs, like white flour, white sugar, and baked potatoes. Best of all, you'll lose weight and keep it off.

Dr. Agatston's diet has produced consistently dramatic results and has become a media sensation in South Florida. Now, you, too, can join the ranks of the fit and fabulous with *The South Beach Diet*.

THE
SOUTH
BEACH
DIET

THE
SOUTH
BEACH
DIET

**The Delicious, Doctor-Designed, Foolproof Plan
for Fast and Healthy Weight Loss**

Arthur Agatston, M.D.

RODALE

NEW YORK

Copyright © 2003 by Arthur Agatston, M.D.

All rights reserved.

Published in the United States by Rodale Books, an imprint of Random House, a division of Penguin Random House LLC, New York.

rodalebooks.com

RODALE and the Plant colophon are registered trademarks of Penguin Random House LLC.

Originally published in hardcover by Rodale, an imprint of Random House, a division of Penguin Random House LLC, New York, in 2003.

Library of Congress Cataloging-in-Publication Data is available upon request.

ISBN 978-0-593-13968-4
Ebook ISBN 978-1-60529-284-7

Printed in the United States of America

Book design by Carol Angstadt

Photographs: © Island Outpost: page 138 (Roger Ruch)

© Michael Katz: pages 144 (Christian Plotczyk), 154 (Michael Wagner), 222 (Michael Wagner), 278 (Christian Plotzyck)

Courtesy of Andre Bienvenue: pages 164 (Andre Bienvenue), 174 (Andre Bienvenue), 226 (Andre Bienvenue)

© Jose Molina: page 206 (Elizabeth Barlow)

© Seth Browardnik/Red Eye Productions: pages 212 (Scott Fredel, J. D. Harris), 268 (Scott Fredel, J. D. Harris)

Courtesy of Michael D'Andrea: pages 234 (Michael D'Andrea), 284 (Michael D'Andrea)

Cover photograph © Hitoshi Kamiizumi/Getty Images

10 9 8 7 6 5 4 3

2020 Rodale Trade Paperback Edition

Dedicated to
my wife, Sari,
for her support,
enthusiasm,
and love

CONTENTS

ACKNOWLEDGMENTS

Writing these acknowledgments is frustrating because it is impossible to mention all those who have supported me and influenced my work. But the research that led to the South Beach Diet was a cooperative effort, and I want to recognize those who directly helped. My prevention research began with coronary artery calcium detection through electron beam tomography (EBT). Dr. Warren Janowitz was, and is, a brilliant and essential partner in this project. David King and Dr. Manuel Viamonte Jr. gave Warren and me great support and advice throughout.

When I decided to work with a diet that defied the conventional wisdom, I went first to Marie Almon, a dietitian, who became an invaluable associate. I received great support and counsel from my colleagues and collaborators Drs. Gervasio Lamas, Eric Lieberman, Charlie Hennekens, Robert Superko, Wade Aude, Francisco Lopez-Jimenez, and Ronald Goldberg.

Kristi Krueger and Jana Ross from WPLG Channel 10 became wonderful partners in bringing the South Beach Diet to the South Florida public.

Finally, when the book project was in doubt, along came author, lecturer, and friend, Linda Richman who connected me with my superb agent, Richard Pine.

THE
SOUTH
BEACH
DIET

PREFACE

When I first developed the South Beach Diet in 1995, my goal was to help my cardiology patients improve their heart health. Word spread quickly through Miami about the weight-loss results my patients were seeing, and a local television station put South Florida on the South Beach Diet. From there, I was encouraged to write a book and share the program with the broader public. I had no idea how far we would come in such a short time. Since its publication in April 2003, *The South Beach Diet* has become an international bestseller that has enabled millions of people to shed unwanted pounds and improve their health. This improvement in the quality of readers' lives has been enormously gratifying, as have been the letters I've received, the e-mails sent to my Web site, and the feedback from people I've met during my speaking trips around the country. I have read and heard many thousands of stories about shrinking waistlines, changed blood chemistries and overall better health.

Just as important as the success of the diet and the difference it's made in people's lives, the principles of the South Beach Diet—good carbohydrates and good fats, nutrient-dense whole foods, lean sources of protein and plenty of fiber—are now widely recognized by doctors and health experts as the basis of a proper diet, one that we should be eating the world over. This is great news, because it means the public will no longer be deluged with conflicting and confusing advice about what to eat. This consensus could not have come at a better time, since the epidemic of obesity and diabetes continues unabated in the United States and is fast becoming a global epidemic as well. (To give you a few examples, one-third of the population of New Delhi is overweight, diabetes is becoming alarmingly common in Beijing, and fast food and processed foods have penetrated Europe, leading to an increase in childhood obesity.)

One fact has become clear to me: while Americans are overfed, we are also dangerously undernourished. Malnutrition has always been associated with images of thin, emaciated souls, but it is now apparent that both overweight and non-overweight Americans are also often malnourished due to the lack of good carbohydrates such as whole vegetables and fruits in their diets, as well as the near absence of the healthy fats like omega-3 oils This is particularly true for children, whose diets are too often based predominantly on refined starches, simple sugars and trans fats, which are the worst kind of fats. I believe that much of the alarming increase in childhood asthma and Attention Deficit Disorder, as well as numerous other maladies, is nutritionally based. Because we have not yet learned to effectively extract the nutrients and vitamins from fruits and vegetables, supplements cannot be counted on to replace nutritious whole foods. What this means is that even for those of ideal weight, following the principles of the South Beach Diet is fundamental for general health.

The challenge today is not to determine the principles of healthy eating, but to find the best methods to implement what we already know. For this, it is necessary to educate health-care professionals as well as the general public. Another factor in changing the way Americans eat is making healthy eating convenient and satisfying. I invite the restaurant, hotel, and food industries to work hard to meet America's desire for healthier, more nutritious foods.

While millions of people have successfully incorporated the South Beach Diet into their lifestyles, there are persistent misconceptions concerning the diet, many of which are communicated by people who have not read the book. First, the South Beach Diet is often identified as a "low carb" diet. While the South Beach Diet is low in processed and refined carbs, it's not a low-carb diet in that it encourages the consumption of the "good cards" that are so important in maintaining our general health and sustaining long-term weight loss. In fact, the South Beach Diet can even be a high-carbohydrate diet, as long as you are choosing the right carbs. The vegetarian version of the South Beach Diet is an example of a high-carbohydrate, healthy diet.

Another misconception is that the South Beach Diet is a high-fat, high-protein diet. From day one, the South Beach Diet has been a low saturated fat diet. We encourage people to eat the "good fats" that are essential for general health as well as preventing heart disease and cancer. The "bad fats"—

the saturated and trans fats—are empty calories that promote heart disease and diabetes. Sources of healthy omega-3 fats are fish, fish-oil supplements, flaxseed, flaxseed oil, and green, leafy vegetables. Range-fed meat as well as poultry and eggs from range-fed poultry are also good sources of omega-3 fats, and they are generally lower in saturated fats than non-range fed meats.

As far as protein is concerned, the South Beach Diet is flexible and does not require a fixed percentage of protein, carbohydrates, or fats. For young athletes, a high-protein diet is safe and optimal. For older patients with hypertension and compromised kidney function, a low-protein diet is appropriate. Both high- and low-protein eating plans can easily be created using the principles of the diet.

The question of calories has continued to be a point of diet controversy. My view is that while calories absolutely do count, counting calories does not work, especially when poor food choices are being made. Counting calories, carbohydrates, grams of fat or weighing foods makes it difficult to make a healthy diet a lifestyle. Our goal is long-term weight loss and health maintenance, not short-term weight loss. This is easy to do without constant counting and weighing, by eating a great variety of healthy, nutrient-rich foods.

Some have suggested that the South Beach Diet should have put a greater emphasis on exercise. My belief in the important role of exercise in general health maintenance and weight control has always been strong and remains so. As I say in part one of the book, some form of regular aerobic exercise, strength training, and stretching, even in short doses, is essential. Short sessions may not necessarily burn lots of calories each time, but will burn enough per year to translate into many pounds. Of equal importance, regular exercise can help build and maintain muscle and bone mass, which otherwise tends to diminish with age. Muscle and bone mass are important determinants of our basal metabolic rate, which dictates the number of calories we burn while resting. The important thing is to choose an exercise program that can become a long-term habit.

I am often asked about the South Beach Diet and children. I have been very gratified to hear the success stories of those who have successfully applied the principles of the diet to the meals the whole family eats. I do want to emphasize that it is not necessary for children to be on a structured diet. What kids need, just as we all do, is to consume more fruits, vegetables, whole grains and good fats, while minimizing their intake of trans fats and simple sugars. If this is accomplished, better health and optimal weight will follow. The earlier children are exposed to healthy choices, the better.

In closing, I want to thank everyone whose success on the diet has contributed to our ultimate goal of changing the way America eats. For those of you who are new to the program, I wish you the best of luck.

Arthur Agatston, M.D.
December 2004

PART ONE

Understanding the South Beach Diet

LOSING WEIGHT, GAINING LIFE

The South Beach Diet is not low-carb.

Nor is it low-fat.

The South Beach Diet teaches you to rely on the right carbs and the right fats—the *good ones*—and enables you to live quite happily without the bad carbs and bad fats. As a result, you're going to get healthy and lose weight—somewhere between 8 and 13 pounds in the next 2 weeks alone.

Here's how you'll do it.

You'll eat normal-size helpings of meat, chicken, turkey, fish, and shellfish.

You'll have plenty of vegetables. Eggs. Cheese. Nuts.

You'll have salads with real olive oil in the dressing.

You'll have three balanced meals a day, and it will be your job to eat so that your hunger is satisfied. Nothing undermines a weight-loss plan more than the distressing sensation that you need more food. No sane eating program expects you to go through life feeling discomfort. You'll be urged to have snacks in the midmorning and midafternoon, whether you need to or not. You'll have dessert after dinner.

You'll drink water, of course, plus coffee or tea if you wish.

For the next 14 days you *won't* be having any bread, rice, potatoes, pasta, or baked goods. No fruit, even. Before you panic: You'll begin adding those things back into your diet again in 2 weeks. But for right now, they're off-limits.

No candy, cake, cookies, ice cream, or sugar for 2 weeks, either. No beer or alcohol of any kind. After this phase you'll be free to drink wine. It's beneficial for a variety of reasons. Not a drop during the first 2 weeks, however.

Now, if you're the kind of person who lives for pasta or bread or potatoes, or if you believe that you can't get through a day without feeding your sweet tooth (three or four times), let me tell you something: You're going to be shocked at how painlessly 2 weeks will pass without these foods. The first day or two may be challenging; but once you weather that, you'll be fine. It's not that you'll have to fight your urges—during the first week the cravings will virtually disappear. I say this with such confidence only because so many overweight people who have already succeeded on this program tell me so. The South Beach Diet may be new to you, but it has existed for several years—long enough to have helped hundreds of people lose weight easily and keep it off.

So that's Phase 1, the strictest period.

After 2 weeks of that, you will be somewhere between 8 and 13 pounds lighter than you are today. Most of that weight will come off your midsection, so right away you'll notice the difference in your clothes. It will be easier to zip your jeans than it's been for some time. That blazer will close without a bulge.

But this will be just the noticeable difference. You won't be able to see that during those 2 weeks you'll also have changed yourself internally. You will have corrected the way your body reacts to the very foods that made you overweight. There's a switch inside you that had been turned on. Now, simply by modifying your diet, you'll have turned it off. The physical cravings that ruled your eating habits will be gone, and they'll stay away for as long as you stick with the program. The weight loss doesn't happen because you're trying to eat less. But you'll be eating fewer of the foods that created those bad old urges, fewer of the foods that caused your body to store excessive fat.

As a result of *that* change, you will continue losing weight after the 14-day period ends, even though by then you will have begun adding some of those banished foods back into your life. You'll still be on a diet, but if it's bread you love, you'll have bread. If it's pasta, you'll reintroduce that. Rice or cereal, too. Potatoes. Fruit will definitely be back.

Chocolate? If it makes you feel good, sure. You will have to pick and choose which of these indulgences you permit yourself. You won't be able to have all of them, all the time. You'll learn to enjoy them a little differently than before—maybe a little less enthusiastically. But you will enjoy them again soon.

That's Phase 2.

You'll remain in that phase and continue losing weight until you reach your goal. How long it takes depends on how much you need to lose. In Phase 2 people lose, on average, a pound or two a week. Once you hit your target, you'll switch to an even more liberal version of the program, which will help you to maintain your ideal weight.

That's Phase 3, the stage that lasts the rest of your life. When you get to that point, you'll notice that this plan feels less like a diet and more like a way of life. You'll be eating normal foods, after all, in normal-size portions. You can then feel free to forget all about the South Beach Diet, as long as you remember to live by its few basic rules.

As you're losing weight and altering how your body responds to food, a third change will be taking place. This one will significantly alter your blood chemistry, to the long-term benefit of your cardiovascular system. You will improve invisible factors that only cardiologists and heart patients worry about. Thanks to this final change, you will substantially increase your odds of living long and well—meaning you will maintain your health and vitality as you age.

You may start on the South Beach Diet hoping just to lose weight. If you adopt it and stay with it, you will surely accomplish that much. But you'll also do a lot more for yourself, all of it very good. I'm not exaggerating when I say that this diet can, as a fringe benefit, save your life.

GOOD CARBS,
BAD CARBS

I'm not a diet doctor.

In fact, my career in medicine has been largely devoted to the science of noninvasive cardiac imaging—the development of technology that produces sophisticated pictures of the heart and the coronary blood vessels. This allows us to identify problems and treat them early, before they cause heart attack or stroke. In CT (computerized tomography) scanning all over the world, I'm proud to say, the measure of coronary calcium is called the Agatston Score, and the protocol for calcium screening is often referred to as the Agatston Method. I maintain an active, full-time cardiology practice, both clinical and research.

So how is it that I am also responsible for a weight-loss program that has become a phenomenon here in South Florida, a regimen that's helped countless women and men—many of them in their twenties and thirties, young enough to be the grandchildren of my usual cardiology patients—get down to string-bikini and Speedo-swim-trunks-shape?

I have to admit, I wasn't prepared to find myself on the receiving end of so much buzz. I'm now regularly stopped by people who have seen my TV news appearances or read about the diet's success in newspapers and mag-

6

azines. Given this city's worldwide image as a mecca of physical beauty and body consciousness and its role as a chic outpost of the fashion industry, it's an unexpected position in which to find myself.

This all started as a serious medical undertaking. Back in the mid-1990s I was but one of many cardiologists who had grown disillusioned with the low-fat, high-carbohydrate diet that the American Heart Association recommended to help us eat properly and maintain healthy weight. None of the low-fat regimens of that era seemed to work reliably, especially over the long haul. My concern was not with my patients' appearance: I wanted to find a diet that would help prevent or reverse the myriad of heart and vascular problems that stem from obesity.

I never found such a diet. Instead, I developed one myself.

Today, I feel nearly as comfortable in the world of nutrition as I do among cardiologists. I speak regularly before physicians, researchers, and other health-care professionals who devote their lives to helping patients eat sensibly and lose weight. Although my interest in diet started from the therapeutic perspective, I see now that the cosmetic benefits of losing weight are extremely important because they so effectively motivate the young *and* the old—even more than the promise of a healthy heart, it often seems. The psychological lift that comes from an improved appearance benefits the entire person, and keeps many a patient from backsliding. The end result is cardiovascular health—my only goal when this journey began.

What started as a part-time foray into the world of nutrition has led me to devise a simple, medically-sound diet that works, without stress, for a large percentage of those who try it. This program has been scientifically studied (as few diets ever are) and proven effective, both for losing weight and for getting and keeping a healthy cardiovascular system.

Back when this all began, of course, I had no idea what would ensue. All I knew was that many of my patients—more of them every year—were overweight and that their condition was a big part of their cardiac risk. I could treat them with all the newest medications and procedures, but until they got their diet under control we were often fighting a losing battle. Their eating habits contributed to blood chemistry that was dangerously high in cholesterol and triglycerides, the leading factors in blocked arteries and inflammation of the blood vessels. And there was another, not terribly well-understood diet-related problem that they shared, a silent, so-called *metabolic* syndrome (prediabetes) found in close to half of all Americans who suffer heart attacks.

Searching for the Right Weight-Loss Plan

My journey to disease prevention through diet actually began when my education as a cardiologist did, 30 years ago. During my training in the late 1970s, I looked forward to treating patients with heart disease—despite the fact that we didn't have many preventive weapons in our arsenal. I asked the most respected cardiologist I knew this question: "What is the best way to prevent heart disease?" His answer: "Pick the right parents." If you inherited the gene for cardiac longevity, you were likely to live to a ripe old age. If heart disease struck early in your family, there was not much you could do to change your destiny.

Then, in 1984, I attended a course at the Heart House in Bethesda, Maryland, the national headquarters of the American College of Cardiology. There, I heard a lecture by a brilliant researcher and charismatic teacher, Bill Castelli, who headed the world-famous Framingham Heart Study. Dr. Castelli told us about the results of the recently completed National Institutes of Health (NIH)–sponsored Lipid Research Clinics Primary Prevention Trial (LRCPPT). This was the very first study to prove that lowering cholesterol could reduce heart attacks. At the time, the only known treatment for high cholesterol was an unpleasant, grainy powder known as a resin, which was taken several times a day before meals. Therefore, we were all very excited when Dr. Castelli told the conference that if we put patients on the very first American Heart Association diet, we could lower their cholesterol and end the scourge of heart disease in America.

We all returned home filled with fervor, ready to guide our patients to restored cardiac health and dietary wisdom. I came back to Miami confident in my newfound knowledge of how to save my patients' lives. My wife and I even joked that with heart disease out of the picture, I might be better off switching to a growth specialty, like plastic surgery. It wasn't long before I learned that unemployment as a cardiologist was going to be unlikely.

I began counseling my patients on the low-fat, high-carbohydrate diet advocated by the American Heart Association, but the results fell far below my expectations. Often, there was an initial modest improvement in total cholesterol with mild weight loss. This invariably was followed by a return of cholesterol to its previous level or higher, along with a return of the lost weight. This scenario was not only my experience but also that of my colleagues. It was reflected in the many diet-cholesterol trials documented in the literature: we were unable to sustain cholesterol and/or weight reductions using low-fat, high-carbohydrate diets. There were no convincing studies showing that the American Heart Association diet saved lives.

Over the years I had suggested most of the highly respected diets out there—going back to Pritikin and then through the various, more recent, heart-healthy low-fat regimens, including the Ornish plan and several American Heart Association diets. Each of them, for different reasons, failed miserably. Either the diets were too difficult to stick with, or the promise of improved blood chemistry and cardiac health remained just that—a promise. Discouraged, I had all but given up on advising my patients about nutrition, because I was unable to suggest anything that actually helped. Like most cardiologists in that period, I turned instead to the statin drugs that were just entering the market, medications that had proven extremely effective in lowering total cholesterol, if not weight.

But I also decided, as a last-ditch effort, that I would devote some serious study of my own to diet and obesity. Like most physicians, I was not particularly knowledgeable in the science of nutrition. So my first task was to research all the weight-loss programs out there, the serious scientific ones as well as the trendy attempts that topped the best-seller lists. As I acquired that education, I was also reading in the cardiology literature about the prevalence of something called the insulin resistance syndrome and its effect on obesity and heart health.

The Science of Success

One side effect of excess weight, we now know, is an impairment of the hormone insulin's ability to properly process fuel, or fats and sugars. This condition is commonly called insulin resistance. As a result, the body stores more fat than it should, especially in the midsection. Since the dawn of *Homo sapiens*, we've been genetically conditioned to store fat as a survival strategy to see us through times of famine.

The problem now, of course, is that we never experience the famine end of that equation, only the feast. As a result, we store fat but never require our bodies to burn it off. Much of our excess weight comes from the carbohydrates we eat, especially the highly processed ones found in baked goods, breads, snacks, and other convenient favorites. Modern industrial processing removes the fiber from these foods, and once that's gone their very nature—and how we metabolize them—changes significantly for the worse.

Decrease the consumption of those "bad" carbs, studies showed, and the insulin resistance starts clearing up on its own. Weight begins a fairly rapid decrease, and you begin metabolizing carbs properly. Even the craving for carbs disappears once you cut down on their consumption. Finally, cutting out processed carbs improves blood chemistry, ultimately resulting in lowered triglycerides and cholesterol.

So my eating plan's first principle was to permit good carbohydrates (fruits, vegetables, and whole grains) and curtail the intake of bad carbohydrates (the highly processed ones, for the most part, where all the fiber had been stripped away during manufacturing). We would thereby eliminate a prime cause of obesity. This was in marked contrast to the Atkins Diet, for instance, which bans virtually *all* carbohydrates and leaves the dieter to exist mostly on proteins. That regimen also permits limitless saturated fats, the kind found in red meat and butter. These are, as most people know, the bad fats—the ones that can lead to cardiovascular disease, heart attack, and stroke. That hasn't stopped millions of dieters from adopting the plan. But from the moment I learned of it, the diet set off alarm bells in this cardiologist's head. Even if you do lose weight and keep it off, your blood chemistry might suffer from eating so much saturated fat.

My plan cut certain carbohydrates, but not all of them. In fact, it encouraged eating the good ones. For instance, I banished white flour and white sugar. But our diet permits whole grain breads and cereals and whole wheat pasta. We also prescribe lots of vegetables and fruits. I had a practical reason for that decision, beyond their obvious nutritional value and the beneficial fiber they provide. Not everyone *wants* to give up vegetables, fruit, bread, and pasta forever, even in exchange for a regimen that allows a pound of bacon for breakfast, followed by a pound of hamburger (with no bun, of course) for lunch, topped by a thick steak for dinner. And if people want bread, pasta, or rice, a humane eating plan should be able to accommodate that desire.

To make up for the overall cut in carbohydrates, my diet permitted ample fats and animal proteins. This decision flew in the face of the famous diets that had been developed specifically for people with heart problems, like Pritikin and Ornish. For a cardiologist, this was skating on thin ice. But my experience with patients showed that those so-called heart-healthy diets were nearly impossible to stick to, because they relied too heavily on the dieters' ability to eat superlow fat over the long haul. The South Beach Diet would permit lean beef, pork, veal, and lamb.

The low-fat regimen's severe restrictions on meat were unnecessary—the latest studies had shown that lean meat did not have a harmful effect on blood chemistry. Even egg yolks are good for you contrary to what we once believed. They're a source of *natural* vitamin E and have a neutral-to-favorable effect on our balance between good and bad cholesterol. Chicken, turkey, and fish (especially the oily ones such as salmon, tuna, and mackerel) were recommended on my diet, along with nuts and low-fat cheeses and yogurt. As a rule, low-fat prepared foods *can* be a bad idea—the fats are replaced with carbs, which are fattening. But low-fat dairy products such as cheese, milk, and yogurt are exceptions to this rule—they are nutritious and not fattening.

I also allowed plenty of healthy mono- and polyunsaturated fats, like the Mediterranean ones: olive oil, canola oil, and peanut oil. These are the good fats. They can actually reduce the risk of heart attack or stroke. In addition to being beneficial, they make food more palatable. They're filling, too—a major consideration for a diet that promises that you won't have to go hungry.

Next, I found a suitable guinea pig for preliminary testing purposes, a middle-age man who was having trouble keeping his growing paunch under control: me. I went on the diet. I gave up bread, pasta, rice, potatoes. No beer. Not even fruit, at least in the very beginning, because it contains high levels of fructose, or fruit sugar. But otherwise I was determined to eat as normally as possible, meaning three meals a day plus snacks when I was hungry.

After just a week, I noticed a difference. I lost almost 8 pounds in those first 7 days, and it was easy. I didn't suffer any hunger pangs. No terrible cravings. No noticeable deprivation.

Almost sheepishly, I approached Marie Almon, M.S., R.D., chief clinical dietitian at our hospital, Mount Sinai Medical Center in Miami Beach, and told her of my experiment. She conceded that the low-fat diet we had been recommending to cardiac patients wasn't working. So we took the basic principles I had developed and expanded them into an agreeable eating plan.

Practical Solutions

We settled on a few more guidelines, based on my clinical experience and study of the literature. First, we acknowledged the primary failing of diets we had tried with patients: They're too complicated and too rigid. A diet may be medically or nutritionally sound, but if it is hard to live with, if it doesn't take into account how the whole person operates—not just his or her digestive tract and metabolism—then it is a failure. So this diet would be flexible and simple, with as few rules as possible. It would allow people to eat the way they actually *like* to eat, while improving their blood chemistry and helping them to lose weight and maintain the loss over the long run. This means a lifetime, not 3 months or a year. Only by accomplishing these goals would this program make the crucial transition from being a diet to being a lifestyle—a way of living and eating that normal human beings can sustain for the rest of their lives.

With that in mind, we decided that we wouldn't ask people to deny themselves every eating pleasure indefinitely. Typically, once you've gone off track on a diet, you're on your own. The experts never allow for human frailty or tell you how to accommodate the inevitable slips as part of the plan. As a result, people who cheat a little today usually cheat a little more tomorrow, and then it's a slippery slope down to where the diet's in shambles, you've broken every rule, and you're depressed, discouraged, and back at square one. So we make ample use of desserts devised especially by Marie Almon for the program. These treats are delicious, yet use only "legal" ingredients.

We also simply recognized that there will be days when you just *need* that chocolate ice cream or lemon meringue pie. I'm a chocoholic, so believe me, I understand. This plan would allow dieters to bend or break the rules, so long as they understood exactly what damage they've done and how to undo it. If the cheating put a few pounds on, or stalled the weight loss, the setback would be minimal and easily repaired, rather than spelling doom. One beauty of the three-phase structure of the South Beach Diet is that you can move easily from one stage to another. If, while in Phase 2, you go on vacation and overindulge in sweets, it's easy to switch back to Phase 1 for a week, lose the weight those desserts put on, and then return to where you left off in Phase 2.

Finally, people are practical beings. Diets that require complex menus, or supplements taken at certain times of day, or foods eaten in precise combinations, are just too burdensome to sustain for long. Many popular diets are extremely tricky in that regard, despite the fact that there is no basis in science for such complexity. And so they fail. Most of us lead complicated enough lives without having to be within walking distance of a refrigerator every 2 hours. Nobody wants to carry around a pillbox or a rule book (or both). So this diet would be based on dishes that are easy to make, with ingredients that are commonly found in supermarkets or in most restaurants. The plan requires snacks between meals, but the kind that can be thrown into a briefcase or backpack in the morning and eaten on the run. Our diet is also distinguished by the absence of calorie counts; percentage counts of fats, carbs, and proteins; or even rules about portion size. Our major concern is that dieters eat good carbs and good fats. Once that's all under control, portions and percentages take care of themselves. By choosing the right carbs and the right fats, you simply won't be hungry all the time.

Our diet, we decided, would have to be effective regardless of the dieter's exercise habits. Without a doubt, exercise does increase the body's metabolism, thereby making the diet more efficient. It is also a critical part of any cardiac health plan. However, the South Beach Diet does not depend on exercise in order to work. You'll lose more weight, faster, if you are active on a regular basis. But you'll lose weight even if you're not.

Flexibility and common sense, guided by real science—as opposed to the pop science that often passes for nutrition these days—were the guiding principles of the South Beach Diet. We hoped we had come up with a workable, practical solution to the obesity that plagued so many people we saw in the office and hospital setting. We believed it would work for most of them. But of course, we wouldn't really know until they tried it.

MY SOUTH BEACH DIET

KAREN G.: I'VE LOST 30 POUNDS AND KEPT IT OFF.
I had just moved back to Miami Beach from Arizona after getting a divorce. And, of course, everybody in that situation goes on what I call the Divorce Diet—you know, you're going to be dating people for the first time in a long, long time. And those 30 extra pounds you put on during 30 years of marriage? Back when you thought it didn't matter?

Anyway, I read about the South Beach diet in the newspaper and it sounded easy, so I got all the details. My big thing is that I hate feeling hungry. I just don't like the sensation. In the past, I had been on plenty of low-fat diets, and I *always* felt hungry. On this diet, though, the rule is that if you feel hungry, you eat. When you sit down to a meal, you're supposed to eat until you're satisfied.

Salty and starchy things were always my weakness, much more than sweets—potato chips, french fries, popcorn. I would go to Target and the first thing I bought was a large bag of popcorn, and by the time I was through shopping it was finished. And I never went to a movie without having buttered popcorn—never, ever, *ever*. I had a husband who wanted dinner from soup to nuts, every night: Salad, meat, potatoes, a vegetable, bread—always bread. For me to sit down in a restaurant and not have bread and butter was a big sacrifice. You know, on most diets they say you can have the bread but not the butter. On this diet you can have the butter, but not the bread. Or if you have the bread, it's whole grain dipped in olive oil instead of slathered with butter.

It wasn't so easy for me in the first few weeks, during the strict phase. I had to cut out all the things I loved—bread, potatoes, rice, pasta, potato chips. I actually didn't feel so great. I felt . . . not bad, exactly, but not completely myself either. For the first 3 weeks I felt like I was getting all that bad stuff out of my system. And while I never was hungry, I still craved all the things I couldn't have.

I don't even have the desire for them now, though. The cravings went away. Now when I want a salad I can have it—and with dressing on it. *Real* dressing, not some crappy stuff that tastes horrible.

My mother went on the diet when she saw the weight I lost. She's 81 and she's got terrible cholesterol, too. After the first couple of weeks she said, "You know, I'm really feeling hungry." And I said to her, "Mom, the point of this diet is that you don't *have* to be hungry. *Eat.* If you're hungry, go get a piece of cheese." She had assumed that if it's a diet, you're supposed to be hungry. She took my advice and started eating, and she still lost about 15 pounds, which she had never been able to take off before.

I'm pretty born again about this diet. I don't cheat a lot. No pasta at all. No rice at all. I can have brown rice, but I don't like it. No potatoes, except for sweet potatoes, and even then, only baked. And not so often. No sweets. I *have* added bread back, because I still love it. Not every day—maybe two or three times a week. And never white. I'll have whole wheat, or rye, or pumpernickel, but even then I always ask if there's any white flour in it. Because many times, there *is*. Rye bread you buy at the supermarket has white flour in it, for instance. So you have to watch it.

Honestly, the best part about this program is that there isn't a restaurant that I can't go into. For lunch, just about any restaurant can make you a salad with vegetables and cheese or meat or fish in it. You can get chicken salad or tuna salad anywhere, too. I can go to Burger King and get a grilled chicken sandwich and throw away the bread. I go to an Italian restaurant that fixes me veal parmigiana without the breading—just tomato sauce and cheese on top. We'll go to a steak house and I'll have shrimp cocktail and steak with a vegetable—steamed asparagus or green beans, and I can put butter on it, too. I don't overdo it, but it's real butter. And I'll have a salad with blue cheese dressing. And that's not cheating!

I went on the diet 3 years ago and I've lost 30 pounds and kept it off. I feel comfortable again. I'm a size 12 now, and I feel fine the way I am. I would love to lose another 10 pounds, but I'm not going to kill myself to do it. I *was* wearing a size 16. So I had to go to the fat-lady store. It's not fun to go to the fat-lady store. ■

A BRIEF HISTORY
OF POPULAR DIETS

I f you're confused about weight-loss programs, you're not alone. At any given moment, popular diets run the gamut from low fat–high carb to high fat–low carb. Some emphasize high protein. Others require precise combinations of nutrients in each meal. In my medical practice, I've found that a good understanding of the thinking behind a diet leads to high compliance. With that in mind, I'll try to give you a basic grasp of the principles of the South Beach Diet.

First, a brief history, to bring you up to speed.

The modern era of better health through weight loss begins with the American Heart Association diet recommendations that grew out of post–World War II studies done by a pioneering researcher, Dr. Ansel Keys of the University of Minnesota. He compared diet to heart attack rates in countries around the world, and found that where there was low intake of fat, people enjoyed better cardiovascular health. This was for the most part true, and it furthered our understanding of how food affects our health.

But it was not entirely true, and it has taken us many years to complete our knowledge of how nutrition and health (especially cardiac health) are connected.

When Dr. Keys performed his studies of the relationship between fat intake and heart disease, he found an exception on the Greek island of Crete, where there was high intake of fat and yet very low heart attack rates. It ran counter to everything else his studies indicated, and so the Crete exception was discounted. This turned out to be an unfortunate decision.

It was largely on the basis of Dr. Keys's findings and other similar studies that national recommendations to lower total fat intake were determined. It was decided at the time not to perform a multi-million-dollar study that would test the effects of a low-fat diet. Instead, the guidelines were set on the basis of the best evidence available. To be fair, it is difficult to measure the long-term effects of diet on the cardiovascular system. Arteriosclerosis builds up in blood vessel walls for a lifetime before it is serious enough to cause heart attack or stroke. Thus, the ideal diet study would have taken many years to complete, during which time the cost of monitoring study participants could be prohibitive.

There was also a political component to the low-fat guidelines—a kind of "nutritional correctness" not unlike the political correctness of recent years. The role that a Senate committee chaired by George McGovern played in the writing of our national dietary guidelines was brilliantly documented by journalist Gary Taubes in the journal *Science* in March 2001. The McGovern committee was originally chartered to fight malnutrition, but in the 1970s it switched to a new goal—the prevention of overnutrition. The campaign started with a preconceived notion: Fat was inherently bad, and our overindulgence in it was the major cause of obesity and heart disease in the United States. The committee also tended to suspect that those who did not believe that fat was Public Enemy Number One were being unduly influenced by the beef, egg, or dairy industry. The bottom line is that low total fat, high carbohydrate became the orthodoxy, despite the lack of proof that such a diet would improve overall health.

Fats versus Carbs: The Debate

How has America done since the low-fat, high-carbohydrate diet recommendations? We've gotten fatter and fatter. In addition, adult-onset diabetes, a sure sign of unhealthy blood chemistry, has become widespread. What went wrong? First, it was thought that the new low-fat American diet would mimic the low-fat, high-carb regimen of countries like China and Japan, which had very low heart attack rates. But the U.S. food industry stepped in to provide us with low-fat foods that tasted good. It created delicious, highly processed foods including cookies and baked goods prominently (and accurately) advertised as low fat, no cholesterol. This is the source of the "empty calories" nutritionists decry. In whole foods, the sugars and starches are bound up with the fiber and nutrients, so when we eat whole grain rice, we get the entire package. Processing removes the fiber (and hence, the nutrients) in order to make that rice easier and faster to cook. But as a result, all we get is the starch, and the calories—empty of the necessary fiber and nutrients.

In addition, the U.S. Department of Agriculture's (USDA) diet pyramid was built on a base of the so-called "complex carbohydrates"— bread, pasta, rice. Like most Americans, I took that to mean that I could eat these foods in abundance and still live thin, healthy, and happily ever after. I was taught in medical school that the only bad effect of sugars was tooth decay. If you recall the '70s, you remember how bread, pasta, and rice were made to seem healthy when compared to the supposed evils of meat.

What have we learned since those days? A lot. First, the concept of dietary fiber as an important component of our nutrition was unknown at the time of Ansel Keys's studies. We didn't begin to appreciate the critical role of fiber until the 1970s. Even then, most of the attention was on fiber's effect on colon and bowel function. In 1980, Dr. Keys wrote a book summarizing his studies; in it, he suggests that fiber *may* have been an important variable not included in his earlier work.

It turns out that the United States and the northern European countries with the high fat intake and high heart attack rates also had the lowest levels of fiber in their carbohydrates. By contrast, less-developed countries with high-carbohydrate, low-fat diets had *lots* of fiber in their carbs. In the 1990s, the Harvard School of Nutrition, under the guidance of Dr. Walter C. Willet, looked at the correlation between fiber and heart attack rates. The finding: When people eat high-fiber carbs such as vegetables and un-processed grains and flour, the danger of most dietary fat becomes minimal. Only saturated fat remains a predictor of heart attacks, and even then not a very impressive one.

When the American Heart Association and other national agencies first issued their low-fat recommendations, most of the fat consumed in the United States was the unhealthy, saturated kind. Not much was known about the effects of other fats (olive oil, fish oils, peanut oils, and such). Be-cause even the experts didn't fully understand the role of fat in health, the recommendations were to decrease total fat intake. In response, saturated fat intake *has* decreased substantially. In fact, the total cholesterol of Amer-icans has decreased even as we have gotten fatter. Why? Because we are eating less saturated fat and more of the good fats, our total cholesterol has decreased. But while our bad cholesterol is lower, so is our good choles-terol, the kind that actually improves cardiovascular function. A third fat in our blood—triglycerides—is also higher, another ill effect of obesity. Triglycerides contribute to clogged arteries.

Finally, we've learned more about the differing natures of fats and carbs when it comes to putting on weight. Ounce for ounce, fats have more calo-ries than carbs. We've always known this, but we've misunderstood the sig-nificance. We took it to mean that carbs are less fattening. In reality, the opposite may be true. When we eat fats, we become satiated. As a result, we know when to stop eating. Refined carbs cause rapid changes in blood sugar levels, stimulate further hunger, thereby encouraging overeating and obesity. Again, this was not known at the time when the low-fat, high-carbohydrate approach was adopted.

In the late 1970s, Dr. David Jenkins, of the University of Toronto, in-troduced the concept of glycemic index. This measures the degree to which eating a particular food increases your blood sugar and therefore con-tributes to weight gain. One of the surprising findings was that certain starches such as white bread and white potatoes increase blood sugar levels faster than table sugar does. The best intentions of the USDA and its pyramid turned out to be a diet based on sugars! It is the widespread adop-tion of this way of thinking that has caused the fattening of America. National guidelines that were created to make us thin and healthy actually made us fatter and sicker.

Understanding Popular Diets

What about the popular diets promoted to the general public over the 30 years since those guidelines were published? Initially, most programs followed the low-fat, high-carb orthodoxy. The most popular was the Pritikin Diet. This regimen requires severe total fat restriction. In recent years, Pritikin has liberalized its view of nonsaturated fats. I admire the Pritikin doctors for their commitment to prevention of heart disease, which has included the successful promotion of exercise. But the problem with the Pritikin Diet, which its proponents acknowledge, is that it is hard to follow and requires a tremendous commitment on the part of the patient. Also, the high carbohydrate content of the diet can worsen cholesterol and triglycerides in certain patients. It definitely is not a diet for the general public.

In the early 1970s, Dr. Robert Atkins wrote *Dr. Atkins' Diet Revolution*, which shocked all by advocating the exact opposite of the low-fat gospel. He called for a diet high in saturated fat and low in carbs and was immediately denounced by the medical and nutritional establishment. The criticism was undermined by the fact that the diet seemed to work much better than the low-fat, high-carb American Heart Association diet. It was also attacked in part because Dr. Atkins limited carbs so severely that body fat was broken down for fuel, causing a condition called ketosis. In otherwise healthy overweight or obese individuals, I am aware of no evidence that ketosis is a danger. But it is associated with a decrease of fluid volume and some dehydration, which can be a problem in patients with kidney disorders or those on antihypertensive medications. Overall, however, the specter of ketosis has been overstated.

The major problem I have with the Atkins Diet is the liberal intake of saturated fats. There is evidence now that immediately following a meal of saturated fats, there is dysfunction in the arteries, including those that supply the heart muscle with blood. As a result, the lining of the arteries (the endothelium) is predisposed to constriction and clotting. Imagine:

Under the right (or rather, wrong) circumstances, eating a meal that's high in saturated fat can trigger a heart attack! In addition, after a high-fat meal certain elements in the blood, called remnant particles, persist for longer than is healthy. These particles contribute to the buildup of plaque in the vessel walls. None of this was known at the time Dr. Atkins developed his diet. But we know it now.

These adverse effects do not occur when the unsaturated fats are consumed. This is why we have strongly encouraged the "right fats" in the South Beach Diet. They make the meals taste good while they actually contribute to healthy vessels.

The other major diet phenomenon of recent years has been Dr. Dean Ornish's plan. The Ornish approach is similar to Pritikin's. It calls for severe total fat restriction and liberal consumption of carbohydrates. He also emphasizes exercise and relaxation techniques. In several small studies, he has demonstrated improved vascular health as a result of his diet. The biggest problem that I see in the Ornish approach is one that he readily acknowledges: It is very difficult to follow. Another issue is its restriction of total fats. Most polyunsaturated and monounsaturated fats are good for you and your blood vessels. So why not use them for satiety and to make meals taste better? Also troubling is that in selected patients, the high carb intake can induce the prediabetes syndrome we'll discuss beginning on page 75. Since at least one-quarter of Americans are predisposed to this syndrome, and it is present in more than 50 percent of those who have had heart attacks, it is no small concern. Ornish developed his diet when the deleterious effect of refined carbs was virtually unknown. Today, Dr. Ornish is putting greater emphasis on high-fiber carbohydrates that will not induce prediabetes.

I knew and admired Dr. Atkins *and* Dr. Ornish. They successfully fought conventional wisdom and both contributed to the country's growing focus on heart attack prevention via improved diet and lifestyle. They were criticized for the commercial success of their programs but have persevered. Unless someone popularizes the science of nutrition, America will never get its difficulties with obesity and heart disease under control.

It is my purpose to teach neither low fat nor low carb. I want you to learn to choose the right fats and the right carbs. You will learn to enjoy foods that taste good, satisfy your appetite, and don't create hunger hours later. In this manner, you can develop the food plans that are best for you for short-term weight loss, long-term weight maintenance, and optimal health.

MY SOUTH BEACH DIET

ELLEN P.: I LOST 20 POUNDS IN 2½ MONTHS. My oldest daughter's bat mitzvah was coming up, and I wanted to lose some weight—maybe 20 pounds or so.

My whole life I had always been able to eat anything and it never showed. I love sweets. Chocolates. My friends had always been jealous. They would say, "How can you eat so much and still be thin?"

So it was a real shock when I hit 40 and all of a sudden, I started gaining weight. My metabolism changed, I guess. Anyway, I didn't really know much about dieting because I never had to. But when I looked around and saw all the weight-loss plans, I said there's no way I'm going to be super-careful about everything I eat, or drink any of those diet shakes, or any of that. That's why this diet was perfect for me, because I never felt like I had to eat things I didn't like or leave the table hungry.

The hardest thing for me at the very beginning was cutting out all fruit. I love fruit and fruit juice. Plus, I'm home a lot with my three kids, and I'm always giving them snacks. At least twice a week my kids and I would buy slice-and-bake chocolate chip cookies. I used to buy a lot of ice cream, too. I'd sit and have a bowl in the middle of the day. Or I'd have cheesecake. Cookies.

At first I didn't know if I could do it. When someone tells me, "You can't eat this," it's almost like I want it even more. But this diet was actually pretty good from the start. My husband went on it with me, and it became almost like a little competition between us. You're not supposed to, but we weighed ourselves every day.

What I liked about the diet was that you really do lose weight right away, and you feel good about that. You can have lobster and shrimp and steak if you're hungry, and vegetables, and you don't have to limit yourself too much. It wasn't even that difficult giving up the sweets. After a while you don't even crave the stuff. And if I was hungry I'd go have a piece of turkey or something. Or cheese. I remember how my husband always had to have his bread. If we went to a restaurant, he would smell bread the second he walked in. Once he went on the diet he would tell the waiter, "Don't even bring it to our table. We don't want to be tempted."

I was on the diet for 2½ months. And in that time I lost 20 pounds. I know you're supposed to stay on the strict phase for only 2 weeks, but I stayed on it a few weeks longer. I wanted to make sure I would lose the weight in time for the bat mitzvah. And even the strict phase wasn't so bad.

I guess I'm on the maintenance phase now. I'm not very strict about it, but I don't crave as much as I did before. I don't even look at ice cream when I go shopping, and I used to want it so much. I used to eat sandwiches all the time, and now I'll have turkey or whatever wrapped up in lettuce instead of bread. I'll cut up leftovers like steak and put them into a salad. Before, I used to skip breakfast most days, but now I always have it, and it seems like that makes it easier to stick with the diet. I'll have an egg with turkey bacon and it satisfies me until lunch. Before, I wouldn't have any breakfast, but if I found some doughnuts I'd have those. I still have cookies once in a while. But that's about it for sweets. ▪

A DAY IN THE LIFE

I started this book by describing, in a nutshell, how you would pass the initial weeks on the South Beach Diet. Now I'll back up and tell you in greater detail how a typical day will go.

Let's start with the first day of Phase 1. You've no doubt treated yourself to a memorable meal the night before, but whatever carb-driven cravings you prompted came as you slept, with no further damage done. By the time you wake up today, your bloodstream is a relatively clean slate. The immediate goal is to *keep* it that way. We will accomplish that simply by not introducing any bad carbs into your system.

We'll begin with a two-egg omelet fortified by two slices of Canadian bacon, cooked in a spray of olive or canola oil. You may yearn for your usual toast or bagel, but if you can get your mind off bread, the rest of you will follow. This will be your first test of the new regimen. It may take a few days to wean yourself from the customary morning dose of carbs. But it's our goal in Phase 1 to begin reversing your body's likely inability to process sugars and starches properly, the condition at the root of most weight problems. To accomplish this, we must cut off all carbs but the healthiest ones. This means we'll allow those highest in fiber and nutrients and lowest in sugars and starches—vegetables and salads only, in other words, at least for these 2 weeks.

This morning's combination of proteins (the eggs and Canadian bacon) and good fats (the oil and the bacon, which is leaner than its American cousin) will keep your stomach full and occupied with digestion. You won't have to contend with hunger pangs now or later this morning. It didn't have to be the Canadian bacon omelet—we could have gone with two eggs and some asparagus, broccoli, mushrooms, or peppers. That would have introduced some good vegetable fiber to the mix. An omelet with ham or low-fat cheese would have been fine, too.

With this meal you can have coffee or tea if you like, with low-fat milk and sugar substitute. There are many to choose from nowadays—I prefer one that's actually derived in part from a form of sugar, although it has no calories. Some diets prohibit coffee or tea because caffeine does intensify cravings somewhat. But you've got enough changes to contend with without having to give up your morning coffee, too.

A phenomenon I've noticed when dealing with overweight people is how many of them skip breakfast altogether—especially women, for some reason. It's not even necessarily an attempt to save on calories. They say they just don't like eating first thing in the morning. The problem is that this allows blood sugar to drop and hunger to increase over the course of the morning, resulting in powerful cravings for a lunch that includes carbs of questionable value—the very kind guaranteed to keep you overweight. So, skipping breakfast is a bad idea, especially if you're trying to fight off obesity.

Planning Your Meals

In part two, we've provided a meal-by-meal, dish-by-dish eating plan for every phase of the diet. As you'll see, the array of breakfasts, even in the strict first phase, is varied. There's a frittata made with smoked salmon, for instance, and something we call Vegetable Quiche Cups to Go, which are made with eggs and spinach and, for the sake of convenience, can be prepared in advance and then microwaved at mealtime. We make liberal use of eggs for breakfast, which will alarm some people who have been taught to avoid them due to cholesterol concerns. It turns out that eggs contain minimal saturated fat and raise the good cholesterol along with the bad. The yolk is a good source of *natural* vitamin E and protein, too. So eggs are permissible. By the second phase of the diet, we'll begin to reintroduce carbs, even whole grain toast and English muffins, along with high fiber cereals. Fruit, too.

Whether you feel the need for a midmorning snack or not, you should be ready for one by 10:30 or so. Wisely, you remembered to pack a part-skim mozzarella stick. As I said in "Good Carbs, Bad Carbs," the only low-fat foods I recommend for dieters are cheese and yogurt, because they're the only ones that don't add bad carbs to replace the fats. The sugar is limited to lactose—milk sugar—which is an acceptable component of the South Beach Diet. You can find cheese sticks in most supermarkets—they've become a favorite snack for children. They're convenient and they taste good. Most important, they do the job of filling you up with good fats and proteins. That means you won't arrive at the lunch hour feeling famished.

When lunch rolls around, you may have a salad—lettuce and tomato mixed with grilled chicken or fish, dressed in a viniagrette made with olive oil. You'll also have water or a beverage containing no sugar. Another day you might choose grilled shrimp over a bed of greens, or a tomato stuffed with tuna salad. Niçoise salad is great, too. All these dishes can easily be made at home, and, thanks to the trend toward fresh, healthy dining out, can usually be found in restaurants, too. Don't even think about limiting the amount you eat—the point of this diet is to eat well. Food is one of life's dependable pleasures, and it can be a wholesome one if you're eating the proper foods. Accomplish that and you'll be free to indulge in the improper treats from time to time.

I hope you are beginning to see the pattern of these meals: They're all combinations of healthy carbohydrates, proteins, and fats. They are normal, everyday dishes intended to fully satisfy your hunger while depriving your system of the low-quality sugars and starches that have wreaked such havoc on your blood chemistry. You may have noticed that we're not discussing calorie counts, fat grams, or portion sizes. The South Beach Diet is designed so that you don't pay attention to any of that. One hallmark of this program is its simplicity—life is complicated enough without having to overanalyze your food before you eat it. If you're eating the right foods you don't need to obsess over how much of them you eat. Since fats and proteins create the sensation of satiety much more efficiently than refined carbs do, you won't sit in front of the TV all night popping bites of steak into your mouth, though you can easily imagine snacking for hours on potato chips or cookies!

By the time you finish this book, you'll have a strong overall grasp of which foods you can eat freely, which you need to enjoy in moderation, and which you'll do without. You'll understand the principles of metabolism—not as a matter of academic interest but in a practical, nuts and bolts way that will give you a basic understanding of how foods affect your blood chemistry and how that, in turn, determines what you weigh. You'll actually learn how to control your blood chemistry and your metabolism through food choices.

Knowing how individual foods affect your internal workings will help you lose weight and maintain the loss. In the future, if you ease up on the diet and find you've gained a few pounds, you'll know how to undo the damage. The glycemic indexes of foods, which are explained and identified on pages 70–74, will be important tools to help you understand which foods contribute to obesity. But once you learn the basics, you'll have all the knowledge you'll need to eat properly. You'll find it easy to cook at home or eat out while sticking to the plan.

Changing Your Thinking

Okay, by now it's midafternoon, typically the first dangerous time of day, dietwise. This is when you might normally crave a sugar fix, owing to the natural dip in blood sugar and consequently, energy, that takes place about this time. This is when people tend to run to the coffee shop, the candy counter, or the vending machines. Instead, you'll have nuts—let's say plain almonds (not salted or smoked). Nuts contain good, healthy fats, and they fill you up. It's possible to have too many of them, however, and undermine your weight loss. I recommend counting out 15 almonds or cashews or whatever you choose. Some people have told me they prefer pistachios, in part because they're so small that you can allow yourself 30 of them. Cracking and eating 30 pistachios makes it a more elaborate, and therefore more satisfying, snack.

Now it's time to begin thinking about dinner. Recent trends in fine food have brought us all toward something close to the South Beach Diet way of thinking—fresh vegetables, fish, and lean meats are the staples of dinner on our program. So Phase 1 features dishes such as grilled salmon with lemon, roasted eggplant and a salad, chicken made with balsamic vinegar, or even marinated London broil and mushroom caps stuffed with spinach. You could happen upon any of these on the menu of a good restaurant and be happy with them. And this is the *strict* phase of the diet! As you'll see in Part II, in the meal plans for Phase 1, we rely on chicken, fish, lean beef, and plenty of vegetables and salads to go with them.

We strongly recommend that you have dessert after that meal. The second dangerous time of day is between dinner and bedtime. This is when all good intentions and strong resolve are challenged. Partly it's just the normal nightly routine—you unwind with a book or in front of the TV, perhaps in the company of friends or family, and the communal snacking habit kicks in. If you've got children, as I do, you've almost certainly got lots of temptations around the kitchen. Or it may just be that you've trained yourself to expect something sweet after a savory dinner.

In any event, we've come up with two basic strategies for dessert during Phase 1. The first, and simplest, is to have some sugar-free gelatin. For people who love fruit, it may even make up for the loss of fresh fruit flavors during these 2 weeks. The other suggestion makes ample use of low-fat ricotta cheese. You can use it as the basis for a number of delicious, permissible desserts. This one is reminiscent of the Italian delicacy known as tiramisu, which combines cheese, chocolate, espresso, and ladyfingers. Instead, you take a half-cup of low-fat ricotta and stir in a few teaspoons of unsweetened cocoa powder, some slivered almonds, and a packet of sugar substitute. It tastes great, and I guarantee that when you're done you'll feel as though you've had a real dessert. We've tried a number of variations on this—using vanilla or almond extract, lemon zest, or even topping the ricotta with sugar-free chocolate syrup and then baking it.

And that's day one on the South Beach Diet! By the time you finish the last bite of mocha ricotta, you will have already begun ridding yourself of the cravings that pushed you into the growing (in every way) ranks of the overweight in America. Your blood is different from the way it was 24 hours ago: it's healthier. Get through another day this way and you'll be even closer to your goal of weight loss, and my goal for you, of better overall health.

MY SOUTH BEACH DIET

DANIEL S.: I FOUND THIS DIET EXTREMELY EASY.
I went to my internist and said I needed a diet. And I said, "I don't want you to give me pills." I'm six-one and I weighed 264 pounds. In my early twenties I was even heavier—probably close to 300 pounds. I lost some of that, but then yo-yoed around with the rest. Physically, I'm in very good shape. Cholesterol, blood pressure, heart—fine. But I was feeling lethargic—unable to move around the way I should.

I go out to dinner a lot. And I was just loading up on a lot of bad things. I am definitely a stress eater, so there were a lot of potatoes and pasta and stuff like that at night. Bread—I soaked it up.

For breakfast, I was always good. Lunch, I tended to be pretty good. It was late afternoon—snacktime—into dinner that was the problem. My afternoon pick-me-up would be a chocolate bar or cookies or something. Clearly not what I should be eating.

And then for dinner—whatever I wanted. I put no limits on myself. Dessert included.

I would say that my downfall was starchy foods. The bad zone was 4 to 8 P.M. An extreme day—a stressful day—would be different starting in the morning. I might have doughnuts or some kind of cake. I'd get an attitude that said: Hey—life's stressful. Might as well enjoy what you can.

I've been on this diet around a year and 2 months now. As I said, I've gone on a hundred diets before this one. A million diets. I've gone from very good results to just moderate. It's very easy for me to lose weight.

It's been nearly impossible for me to keep it off. I'd lose for 4 months, 6 months. And then it would creep back up.

I found this diet extremely easy. I could reintroduce a lot of stuff into my eating after the initial strict phase of the diet. I found that, as we added foods back, I was able to live a fairly normal life, with some modifications of my own. The main thing is teaching myself that, after lunchtime, I cannot put bread, potatoes, or pasta into my system. So that's how I've lived the past year, not eating any of those foods after, say, 5 P.M. I can live without pasta and potatoes. But bread is the one I'm still weak for. And so I've just forced myself to do without it. At a restaurant I ask the waiter not to bring bread to the table. That's not to say I haven't had bread in the last year. But when I have had it—or potatoes or pasta—at night, it shows up as a stall in my weight loss. So there's a clear correlation between those three items and maintaining my weight.

On certain occasions—my birthday, for one, a few weeks ago—I went to a great Italian restaurant, and they made homemade pasta. I had a bowl and I soaked it up with garlic bread. It was phenomenal. But it was my birthday. I should enjoy myself on my birthday. I also had dessert that night. But the next night, and ever since that night, I haven't had any of that stuff.

For lunch or breakfast I'll have a little bread sometimes. Never later than that. And I don't feel denied at all. That's the difference between now and the past. There are times where I see bread and think: Oh, gee, I'd really love a piece. But I've taught myself to go without it. ∎

GOOD FATS, BAD FATS

All fats in our diets were initially condemned due to guilt by association. The dominant fat was saturated fat, and since there was good evidence that this fat was dangerous, all fats were presumed dangerous. To avoid saturated fats in the diet, a special type of polyun-saturated fat became popular: the trans fats. They are the partially hydrogenated oils found in so many commercial products, including cakes, cookies, and margarines. Unfortunately, they are as dangerous, or more dangerous, than saturated fats. They increase bad cholesterol levels and are associated with heart attacks and strokes.

An ever-growing body of research documents that many fats do not have the adverse effects of the saturated and trans fats. In fact, evidence is building that the unsaturated, non–trans fats are actually good for us. Where Mediterranean oils are used abundantly, heart attack and stroke rates are very low.

The most impressive diet study ever reported was the Lyon Heart Study. Here, the mostly monounsaturated fat canola oil (with omega-3 fat as well) was used in a spread by one-half of the patients studied. All those in the study had already had heart attacks, but those receiving the good fat had a 70 percent decrease in subsequent heart attacks.

Another large clinical trial, the GISSI Prevention Trial, showed that fish oil capsules—omega-3 polyunsaturated fats—decreased sudden deaths. Several diet studies have shown that eating fish a few times a week prevents heart attacks and strokes. Omega-3 fat appears to be a major missing ingredient in Western diets.

Finally, a number of studies have documented that several forms of nuts that are rich in mono- and polyunsaturated fats help prevent heart attacks and strokes. This gives us a great variety of foods, oils, and spreads that can make our meals taste great while actually improving our health. So including the right fats in the South Beach Diet was an easy call, and it's looking better and better as more good fat studies are reported.

Once we fine-tuned the diet, it seemed ready for a real test drive. We photocopied the rules plus some basic meal plans and a list of permitted and prohibited foods, along with a few simple recipes. We then began handing them out to our patients. Again, our top priority was *not* weight loss for its own sake—it was to improve our patients' heart health by changing their blood chemistry. We wanted a diet that would lower triglycerides (fats carried in the blood, which are necessary, but when excessive cause serious cardiovascular damage) and LDL (low-density lipoproteins, the so-called bad cholesterol). We were looking for a decrease in LDL both as a total number and as compared to the level of HDL (high-density lipoproteins), the so-called good cholesterol.

And we were also trying to affect one more thing, something that most cardiologists, unfortunately, have yet to give its proper due: the actual size of the LDL particles. When these are small, they easily squeeze beneath the blood vessel linings, narrowing the passageways with a buildup of fatty plaque that eventually leads to heart attack and stroke. Using the right diet, we learned, it is actually possible to increase the size of the LDL particles. As a result, they don't fit under the blood vessel lining as readily, and so won't clog the arteries and cause an emergency somewhere down the line. Most doctors don't test for this crucial factor. In fact, today most blood labs still don't have the equipment required to determine the size of LDL molecules. In the not too distant future, however, measuring for this will become standard operating procedure, as common as cholesterol testing is today.

Our secondary goal, of course, *was* weight loss, because when that occurs it's a sign that blood chemistry is also coming under control. I wasn't thinking that my patients would attain the lean, mean, low-body-fat physical perfection typically associated with this city. And frankly, neither were they.

Almost at once, the patients who went on our diet began to experience positive results. Blood chemistry improved dramatically.

One patient, a man who lives in the Bahamas, came to us in pretty bad shape. Blood work showed high triglycerides, high bad cholesterol, small LDL particles: the triple threat. To make matters worse, he had stubbornly vowed never to exercise—it bored him, he said. And he refused to give up his beloved daily dish of ice cream. With attitudes like that, he was headed for trouble. But on our diet his blood chemistry improved quickly—triglycerides down, bad cholesterol down, good cholesterol up. He never did exercise, either, and he *still* has his daily ice cream. But as a result of the diet he's lost almost 30 pounds, and it's stayed off for 5 years.

Another man was in his mid-fifties when he became my patient. His blood pressure was high, just like his cholesterol and triglycerides, and he already had noticeable narrowing in his coronary arteries. To treat those problems, his previous doctor had prescribed the usual daily cocktail of pharmaceuticals that heart patients everywhere depend upon. We put him on the diet, and before very long his cardiac profile improved. His triglycerides, for instance, had been over 400—frighteningly high. After a month on the diet that number had fallen below 100, a normal level. And he had lost more than 30 pounds, which he's kept off. He's no longer taking all those heart medications.

Another patient should have known better—he is a physician, after all— but he was also an overweight diabetic who had recently begun suffering chest pains. He had undergone one angioplasty to open up an artery, but it had begun to close again. After our first consultation I put him on the diet. His wife did all his cooking, and, understandably, she found it easier to eat what he ate rather than prepare two different dinners every night. She lost weight, too. This particular dynamic has been a pleasant surprise for us—couples losing weight and improving cardiac health together because one of them has to diet. It becomes a shared effort, and they help keep each other on the wagon. In fact, the doctor's wife lost more weight than he did. Between them, they dropped 80 pounds. And before long his blood chemistry normalized. His diabetes resolved, so he no longer requires medication to control his blood sugar and cholesterol. And his arteries stayed clear.

These cardiology patients lost 10, 20, 30, even 50 pounds within months. They started losing as soon as they went on the diet—within the first week. They kept it off, too. Best of all, they reported that the regimen wasn't difficult. The few basic principles were simple and easy to remember, and the rules were flexible. Dieters said they never felt hungry or deprived. After a while they barely noticed that they were dieting.

Most of those patients, male and female, had what we call central obesity—excess weight concentrated around the midsection. We measure waist-to-hip ratio to gauge a patient's pattern of obesity: when the waist is bigger than the hips, it's a warning sign for present or future heart problems. The first part of the body that this diet affects is the waistline—that's where middle-age fat tends to be stored, so that's where the loss is most noticeable. Our patients felt sleeker after just a week or so on the diet. This was very encouraging to the dieters and gave them the inspiration they needed to stick with the program.

After years of prescribing failed diets, I was ecstatic with the results.

Before long, however, there was yet another pleasant surprise. We began getting calls and reports from friends and acquaintances of our patients who had heard about the diet, tried it, and were successfully losing weight. Our patients, we discovered, had begun suggesting the diet to family members, friends, and far-flung relatives. Thanks to e-mail, it was spreading like brushfire. People who had no heart problems at all, even the youngest and most stylish denizens of South Beach, were hearing about the diet, trying it, and shedding pounds. We started handling a steady stream of questions from people we'd never met (long-distance calls in many cases), folks asking what the diet did and did not allow, or requesting recipes and volunteering stories of quick, painless weight loss.

Then, reporters began calling. It's amazing how much space in newspapers and magazines is devoted to weight loss. It's become a spectator sport. In early 1999, we got a call from a news producer at WPLG, the local ABC affiliate TV station. They had heard about us and offered a proposition: They'd find a sampling of Miami Beach residents who wanted to lose weight and put them on our diet. The 6 and 11 P.M. news programs would then track their progress daily over the course of an entire month. We were excited by the idea and confident of the outcome.

The series ran every day—during the sweeps period, when ratings are used to set advertising rates. Hundreds of Miamians went on the diet and lost weight. WPLG also succeeded—the station won the ratings race, moving to first place among nightly news shows, attributed in part to the South Beach Diet project. The station's news director termed it "a huge success with our viewers," and reported receiving hundreds of phone calls and e-mails seeking copies of the plan. The South Beach Diet series became an annual event for the station for 3 years. Our program became a full-fledged municipal endeavor down here. Brochures explaining the diet and the recipes were handed out in Winn-Dixie and Publix supermarkets. They, too, reported high interest and increased sales of the items we recommended.

I've accepted many invitations to discuss our diet at medical meetings where cardiologists and others gather to discuss treatment matters, including prevention and diet. In the beginning, because I am a cardiologist, I expected to be grilled rigorously on my nutritional knowledge. Instead, it became clear that the diet was scientifically sound. Even better, doctors have begun trying the diet themselves and reporting their successes to me. So many doctors have lost weight and improved their blood chemistries on the South Beach plan that it's become known as something of a "physician's diet."

Many of the dieters who came to us through the TV news coverage have been in their twenties and thirties. One young woman, 30 pounds overweight, had been trying to conceive for 7 years. She tried the diet, lost the weight in just a few months, and then discovered she was pregnant. Though we were willing to take credit for this pleasant turn of events, it wasn't until about a year later that I discovered why the diet had allowed her to conceive. There is a condition called polycystic ovary syndrome that is a common cause of abnormal periods and infertility in young women. It turns out that it is due to insulin resistance or prediabetes. By reversing this syndrome with the diet, her periods normalized and a successful pregnancy followed. She is now enjoying her lovely little daughter. Another woman, also in her thirties, an entrepreneur, put her entire company on the program, and they all lost weight together. Many of the nurses here at Mt. Sinai have become familiar with the diet and, almost casually, have begun following it. They often stop me in the hospital corridors to give me updates on their weight loss.

We were encouraged by how easy it is to learn—and put into practice—the operating principles of this program. For example, one of the TV news cameramen reported that he lost weight based solely on the information he picked up in the course of taping my interviews. A couple of years ago, I described the principles behind the diet almost offhandedly to a young colleague at a medical meeting. A year later I was pleasantly surprised to hear he had lost over 50 pounds on the basis of my shorthand explanation. That's become a hallmark of this diet: The basics are easily learned and applied, with no complicated rules, charts, or calculations.

A Proven System

Now it was time to measure our results in a scientific setting. First, we tracked in detail the weight and blood test results of 60 patients who had gone on the diet. The results were very encouraging: Almost all experienced weight loss, lowered triglycerides, lowered LDL cholesterol, raised HDL, and improved waist-to-hip ratio. I presented this initial experience at an NHLBI (National Heart, Lung and Blood Institute) symposium at the annual American Heart Association meeting. The director of the NHLBI acted as moderator of the session. While I was experienced in presenting research at such meetings, it was always in the area of heart imaging, my specialty. Now, I was out of my comfort zone and quite nervous giving a presentation on diet and nutrition. I feared I'd be deluged with hostile questions raising points we hadn't considered. Instead, the very first response from the audience was to congratulate me for having the courage to challenge the American Heart Association's low-fat orthodoxy. It became clear that many of the clinicians in that room had also had discouraging results with recommending low-fat, high-carb diets. I was relieved and very excited that we were on the right track.

We then conducted a study pitting our diet against the strict "step 2" American Heart Association diet. We randomized 40 overweight volunteers to either of the diets, meaning that half went on the Heart Association program and half got the South Beach Diet. None of the subjects knew where their diet had come from. After 12 weeks, five patients on the Heart Association diet had given up, compared to just one on the South Beach plan. South Beach dieters experienced a mean weight loss of 13.6 pounds, almost double the 7.5 pounds lost by the Heart Association group. Our patients also showed a greater decrease in waist-to-hip ratio, suggesting a true decrease in cardiac risk. Triglycerides dramatically decreased for the South Beach dieters, and their good-to-bad cholesterol ratio improved more than that of the Heart Association group. We presented this study at the annual national meeting of the American College of Cardiology, where it was well-received. We've come a long way since the day I decided to act as Test Subject Number One for the South Beach Diet.

At this point, the next step practically suggested itself: It was time to put everything we'd learned into a book and make what has happened here happen across the country.

 MY SOUTH BEACH DIET

MICHAEL A.: I LOST 35 POUNDS IN 4 MONTHS.
I started this diet because my mother had seen a segment about it on the local TV news here in Miami. She has heart disease and was concerned about my health—I was 36 at the time and I weighed about 250 pounds. So as a Father's Day gift she made an appointment with the Mt. Sinai Hospital nutritionist for me.

My food weakness was quantity. I'm not a big sweets person. I would drink a few beers, especially on weekends. That was tough to cut back on. I never ate breakfast, just coffee. For lunch I'd have a salad or pasta. But I snacked all day—whatever they brought into the office, I'd have. Pork rinds. Baked things. And a normal dinner—some kind of meat or fish, with potato or rice or pasta. A lot of high-carb foods. But big portions of everything.

It was even worse on weekends—I'd go out to eat maybe Friday, Saturday, and Sunday, and I'd have a drink or two with dinner. And restaurant food typically isn't the healthiest you can eat. I wasn't exercising at all, either.

When I met with the nutritionist, she said my habits weren't great but they weren't awful, either. It was the combination of what I was eating, and how much of it, and the fact that I wasn't exercising. I had tried diets before, and had lost weight, too. Once I stayed on a diet for 4 months. But when I stopped, all the weight came back.

I finally went on this one, about a year ago, when I weighed more than I ever had. It had gotten to where my clothes no longer fit, and I just was refusing to go out and buy all new clothing. That's when my mother gave me the gift of the nutritionist visit.

The first days weren't so bad. The nutritionist explained to me the initial, strict phase of the diet, and said I could stick with it for 2 to 4 weeks. I'm a real meat eater. So in the initial phase, which allows you unlimited amounts of lean protein, I was all right. What I gave up in carbs I added in meat, so I wasn't hungry. Eggs for breakfast with some ham in there. They told me to cut out the half-and-half with my coffee because of the fat, so I tried the no-carb and nondairy creamers, and I just couldn't do it. That was one area I said I can't cut out. I'll use just a little.

That would pretty much hold me until lunch, which would be a small salad with a decent-size serving of cut-up ham or turkey or chicken. In the afternoon I'd feel hungry, so I snacked on low-fat cheese. I drank a lot of water. Dinner was chicken breast or grilled steak. And that was pretty much it. A small serving of vegetables, but not a lot. I was really trying to cut the carbs. No fruit at all for the first 4 weeks. Only water to drink. During this time, I also started exercising. Three or four times a week I'd walk on a treadmill here at home, 30 to 40 minutes at a time.

I ate the same way on weekends that I did during the week. If I went to a restaurant I'd have a small salad with low-fat dressing and then a steak. No beer, no alcohol, no dessert, no baked potato, no rice. I did the initial phase for 4 weeks instead of the 2 they recommend, because I found it very easy to do and I was seeing results. The Fourth of July came during the first week of my diet. We had people over and they were drinking and having all kinds of good stuff. But I stuck to my diet.

After that first month, I started introducing carbs from the low end of the glycemic index. I'd have bigger salads, and I added some fruit back in, which I had really missed. I began having an apple or a pear after lunch. I found a whole grain bread in the health food section of the local market. It was very low in carbs, and some days I'd have a sandwich on that instead of a salad. I went on vacation that summer and did okay. I stuck to my diet pretty much, didn't gain any weight but didn't lose any either. When I came back home I went back on the strict phase, with exercise, too. On my next visit to the nutritionist we added some more vegetables, like sweet potatoes, wild rice, brown rice, squash, beans, and legumes.

After about 4 months, I was down 35 pounds. My initial goal was a 10 percent weight reduction in 6 months. I got there in 4. My next target was another 10 percent, for a total of 50 pounds lost. From around Thanksgiving to New Year's, I really didn't stay on the diet very strictly. Still, I did okay. I ended up gaining about 7 pounds over the holidays. In January, back to the diet—the strict phase—and exercising.

I've been on this diet almost 8 months. I've never stuck with anything this long. I find it's not hard to do. You can do it when you're on vacation, or when you eat out. It just takes a little discipline and willpower. When people start digging into desserts around me, now and then I'll take a spoonful, too. But I won't have a whole dessert for myself.

I have another 15 or 20 pounds to go. I'm confident that by sometime this year—with exercise and the diet—I'll be there. ▪

HELLO, BREAD

Once you've lasted through the 2 weeks of Phase 1 and rid yourself of your sugar addiction, you are ready to begin adding more carbohydrates to your diet. By this time the insulin resistance syndrome has disappeared. The cravings for sugars and starches are virtually gone, too. It's a fresh start.

You'd think that the challenge would be to restrain dieters from adding too many high–glycemic index carbs too soon, but just the opposite usually happens: People are reluctant to leave the safety of Phase 1 and begin eating the kinds of foods that made them overweight in the first place. If it was bread or rice that made me fat, why would I want to start eating it again? I don't want to undo all the good I've just done. I certainly don't want to slow my weight loss.

Still, there are several good reasons for adding more carbohydrates. First, many are good for you, especially those in fruit. Even bread, if you choose a whole grain type, brings nutritional benefits. Also, it's important for dieters to enjoy their food as much as ever and have a varied array of dishes and ingredients from which to choose. People love to eat, and you can take advantage of that passion even when you can't eat every single thing you want with reckless abandon.

Of course, we add the higher glycemic index carbs slowly. Usually we recommend that you start with one piece of fruit a day, something that won't provoke a big rise in blood sugar. Apples are fine—their glycemic index is low, and there's lots of beneficial fiber in the skin. Grapefruit is another safe choice, as are berries.

At this stage we advise patients *not* to have fruit with breakfast, however. Sometimes it will cause a bigger jolt of insulin if it's eaten first thing in the day, triggering cravings for more. And while whole fruit has lots of fiber, it also contains substantial amounts of fructose—fruit sugar. So save it for after lunch or dinner.

Another carb that can be added back in the early days of Phase 2 is cereal, either something eaten cold, like Kellogg's All-Bran with Extra Fiber, or real (not instant) oatmeal. (The South Beach Diet never requires you to weigh your food. But we'll counsel dieters who are adding rice back into their diets to eat servings no bigger than a tennis ball. And don't choose the biggest potatoes in the supermarket bin.)

In any event, if it's oat bran you want, we suggest that you have it with a sugar substitute and nonfat milk. Adding an egg, which contains protein and good fat, will slow the absorption of the carbs.

If you decide to have your new carbohydrate with dinner instead of breakfast, you can have a slice of whole grain bread at night without fear of doing any damage. But you can't have it at breakfast *and* dinner, at least not in the beginning. Here's the principle to adding more carbs back safely: Do it gradually and attentively. The goal is to eat more carbs again while continuing to lose weight. If you add an apple and a slice of bread a day and you're still dropping the pounds, that's great. If you try having an apple, two slices of bread, and a banana daily and notice that your weight loss has stalled, you've gone too far. It's time to cut back, or try some different carbs and monitor the results.

You'll go on that cautious way as long as you're in Phase 2, eating the most beneficial carbs and paying attention to how they affect you. I'm not talking about weighing yourself every day. I'm actually opposed to that. You can usually tell when you've put on weight, and if you can't your clothes will let you know. You should also be aware of foods that increase cravings.

No two people will experience this phase the same way. Some dieters can have pasta once a week and experience no detrimental effects. Others have to avoid pasta but are all right with a sweet potato. Because we want a diet that's flexible and adaptable to your tastes and habits, you'll have to figure this dynamic out for yourself. Our goal is to help you arrive at a diet filled with foods that you love eating. These rules are sufficient for you to create your own version of the plan.

The most successful dieters, we've found, are the ones who try every recipe imaginable and take advantage of all the foods and ingredients permitted. They make interesting use of herbs and spices—especially the more intensely flavored ones such as horseradish, hot peppers, garlic, cinnamon, and nutmeg. One patient invented a new soup made with every green vegetable he could find.

Boredom is the enemy here. It leads people back to their bad old ways. So at every stage, it's best to make this diet as lively and diverse as possible.

The most effective strategy for achieving your goals is to make use of creative substitutions. This is one of the pillars of this diet—replacing bad carbs with good ones so that you end up eating the things you love, but with slight variations.

We've already discussed the staples: whole grain bread instead of white, sweet potatoes instead of white, brown rice or wild rice instead of white, whole grain pasta. Those substitutions will take you a long way toward making this diet effective. But there are plenty of other tricks.

Here's a terrific one to take the place of mashed potatoes, which everyone loves and, of course, are absolute diet-busters. Instead of potatoes, steam some cauliflower, either fresh or frozen—it makes no difference. (You can even do this in the microwave.) Once it's soft, mash it with a little liquid butter substitute—I Can't Believe It's Not Butter! tastes terrific and has no bad trans fatty acids. Then, mix in a little Land O' Lakes nonfat half-and-half substitute, which also tastes good and is healthy. Salt and pepper to taste, and you've got something that quite honestly can compete any day with the real thing.

Back when we first started the diet, before the trend of "wrap" sandwiches had swept through restaurants, we had some success getting patients to replace bread with lettuce leaves. They'd take sandwich contents—meat or fish, cheese, vegetables, even condiments—and roll them up in crisp lettuce. They found, to their surprise, that the bread wasn't as crucial a part of the sandwich as they had thought it was. The filling was what tasted so good and satisfied their hunger, much more than the bread. We also suggested lots of concoctions that came right out of the '50s—food stuffed inside other food, like tomatoes filled with tuna salad. We had people trying this with any vegetable large enough and strong enough to withstand such treatment: stuffed eggplant, zucchini, and artichokes were big favorites.

We tried a few dessert tricks, too. People who love chocolate almost always love lots of it, but they don't realize how satisfying even smaller amounts can be. Instead of some big chocolate dessert, try strawberries dipped in dark chocolate (which has less sugar than the milk chocolate variety). A few of these and you're satisfied, but in truth you've had a relatively small amount of chocolate and quite a bit more fruit. We also told people to slice bananas, freeze them, and then dip the slices in a sugar-free chocolate sauce. It satisfies any sweet tooth, again, with a small amount of chocolate.

Using the strategy of substitution you can continue eating things that other programs would banish forevermore, including some of the delicacies listed here. First, though, you need to know exactly which ingredients require replacement. The foods and food combinations that follow can, with modifications, support your weight-loss efforts instead of slowing them down.

Bacon and Eggs

Even recently, the prevailing view of nutrition would behold the classic American breakfast of eggs, bacon, home fries, toast, orange juice, and coffee and easily pick out what's unhealthy—the eggs (cholesterol), bacon (fat), and coffee (caffeine)—from what's good for you—the potatoes (a vegetable), bread (nothing's more wholesome than toast, right?) and the OJ (all that vitamin C).

Of course, that view is wrong based on what we know now. That's what can be most frustrating about science: What's praised as good today may be condemned as bad tomorrow, and vice versa. It's not necessarily that we were wrong then and right now. It's just that our knowledge is constantly growing, and along the way we sometimes have to unlearn what we thought was true.

Breakfast is a good example of this. Back before World War II, eggs were considered healthy—high in protein and other nutrients. Then, beginning in the '70s, when doctors first began looking into the ill effects of cholesterol, eggs suddenly became a prime culprit. You were advised to limit yourself to two or three a week, and none at all if you had a high cholesterol. Bacon, too, because of the saturated fats and chemicals used in curing it, was portrayed as not just bad, but toxic. We didn't worry about carbohydrates as a category of food, and especially not about orange juice, which became America's favorite health drink.

We now know that eggs are a perfectly fine food. It turns out that they raise both kinds of cholesterol, the good along with the bad, and they do not adversely affect the ratio of the two—which is the number that really counts. The yolk contains natural vitamin E, an important antioxidant that helps prevent cancer and heart disease.

Even the bacon's not so terrible, so long as you don't overdo it. The coffee's acceptable too, with the same caution.

The rest of the breakfast, though, has got to go. The hash browns? We've already discussed how high the glycemic index of potatoes is, especially the white ones. And when a food is chopped into small pieces, it more rapidly yields its sugars and starches. Take a white potato, cut it into slivers, deep-fry it in some unhealthy oil—it tastes great but wreaks havoc on your blood chemistry.

The toast? You know by now how bad white bread is for anyone trying to lose weight. Each slice is worse than a spoonful of table sugar. If the label on the bread boasts that it's "enriched," you're really in trouble. Manufacturers add nutrients only because the natural ones in the wheat have been removed along with the fiber. People today feel wise when they order whole wheat or rye toast, another triumph of marketing and labeling, because the term whole wheat is almost meaningless. The bread may have more nutrients, but the flour is still highly refined. That label does not signify that you're getting the entire grain of wheat, fiber and all, as you should—that's only in whole *grain* bread. And whole grain bread is rarely found in a supermarket or on a restaurant breakfast table.

Did you decide, for health reasons, to spread your toast with jelly instead of butter? The problem with that decision is that most jellies are loaded with sugar. Butter (within limits) would actually be better for you, since fat slows the absorption of the carbs in the bread. There are better things to eat on bread than butter, but jelly isn't one of them. Same is true for jam. It's loaded with sucrose—table sugar.

How about that orange juice? If it's processed and sold in a carton, you could drink cola with nearly the same results. There are good nutrients in orange juice, but you can get those any number of ways without having to take in all the sugar that comes along for the ride in processed juice. Fresh-squeezed is somewhat better, because it has fiber—the pulp—that slows the absorption of the fructose. We tend to believe that the sweetness of fruit and the sweetness of, say, candy, are two totally different things, but they are not. All the tastes we describe as sweet come from sugars. Fructose, the sugar found in fruit, does in fact have a lower glycemic index than table sugar. Mixed in with fiber, fructose is acceptable. Without the fiber, it can hurt your diet. So eat whole fruit rather than drink juice.

Can you have your favorite breakfast and stick to the South Beach Diet? Yes, with a few modifications.

Cook the eggs in a healthy way, such as boiling or poaching. If you fry, use a spray oil—either soy, canola, or olive—rather than butter or margarine.

Try Canadian bacon instead of the usual kind—it's leaner, lower in saturated fat, and higher in protein than the regular kind.

The potatoes have got to go—there's no way to salvage them. But they can be replaced with cereal, especially oat bran, which has lots of fiber and helps with cholesterol, too. Stay clear of instant oatmeal, however—less fiber, more bad carbs. Get the kind you actually have to cook for a few minutes, the coarser the better, and use a sugar substitute, not sugar, and skim milk (if you require any). Oatmeal may not be an even swap for those good home fries, but it can be an acceptable substitute. Some sacrifices must be made.

If you love the taste of orange too much to give it up, eat the whole fruit. That way you get juice, flesh, fiber, nutrients, vitamin C—the whole package as nature intended. And I'll wager you won't consume three or four oranges at a sitting, the way you do when you drink a big glass of juice.

You can have a slice of whole grain toast, topped with some heart-healthy spread—there are several good ones out there to be found in most supermarket dairy sections. These are not the margarines of old, which contain those bad trans fatty acids that can harm your cardiovascular system.

The coffee is fine, too, with low-fat milk and sugar substitute (if any sweetener).

Nowadays, of course, the classic bacon and egg breakfast is being overshadowed by its fast-food interpretation—the Egg McMuffin. In this meal we have to contend with the bad, saturated fat in the bacon. But the portion of meat is so small that it's not really a major concern, unless you're having two of these every day. As for the egg itself, it's probably not being cooked in the healthiest fat, but again, there's good protein and nutrients without dangerous amounts of bad cholesterol, so even this is permissible. The biggest problem, of course, is in the highly processed carbs in the white-flour muffin. If you have that plus the potatoes and fruit juice, you're having a high–glycemic load start to your day, ensuring cravings for more carbs later. McDonald's is no health food emporium, but then no one who dines there is under any false impression. If you must indulge, either throw away the entire muffin and eat with a fork, or just order the scrambled eggs and bacon breakfast, hold the potatoes, hold the juice.

Banana Split

It seems wholesome, as desserts go, but this one is a killer. Banana is a fruit, true, but like most tropical fruits it has a fairly high glycemic index, up near pineapple and mango. So first we've got to replace it with strawberries or blueberries or raspberries, all of which go just as nicely with ice cream. Along with the fruit, add some nuts—not the kind drenched in sugary syrup, but raw walnuts, almonds, Brazil nuts, or peanuts. They're fine for you and add some bulk and good fat. As for the ice cream itself, there's not much you can do. True, it's loaded with sugar, which is no diet's friend. But it's also loaded with fat, meaning that once you eat it your hunger will be satiated. And you won't be under the delusion that you've been good, so you'll be less likely to think you deserve more tomorrow night. Whereas eating low-fat ice cream or frozen yogurt has none of these advantages—the fat has been replaced with sugar, so it's actually worse for your diet, plus it won't be as satisfying as the real thing, and you might actually convince yourself that you've been virtuous. If you're going to break the rules, you should at least know that you did it.

Cheeseburger

This may be the pinnacle of American cuisine—a cheeseburger, french fries, and a Coke. You can't deny that it's delicious, and thanks to the fast-food empires we've built, it's the easiest meal to come by in the history of eating. It's also highly problematic, though not for the reasons you've been led to believe.

The average fast-food burger itself is something of a health hazard, due to its high saturated fat content and the grease in which it's cooked. Eating one a day is a very bad habit indeed, but as an occasional treat it can be accommodated into the South Beach regimen. However, if instead of this you have a burger in an upscale restaurant, or better yet at home, you begin to change it instantly. You can have a burger made from a good cut of meat, like sirloin, which is much leaner than common ground beef.

But what will you serve that burger on? The usual soft white bun is all sugar. It's improved just by throwing the top half away and eating your meal with a knife and fork. Even better is to have that burger on whole wheat pita or sourdough bread instead of the bun. While sourdough bread is not whole grain, it has another quality that decreases its glycemic index—it is acidic. Acid slows down the stomach's emptying of food into the small intestine, meaning slower overall digestion and slower increase and subsequent decrease in blood sugar.

Best of all—see if you can live without any bread on it.

Next, the ketchup should go—even if you don't use much, it's loaded with sugar. Tomato slices are fine. Lettuce, pickles, and onions are perfect. Mustard's great, and even mayonnaise, as long as you don't overdo it. Remember to use the regular kind, not the low fat. Regular mayonnaise is high in fat, but it is predominantly soybean oil, a good fat. Salsa, hot sauce, steak sauce are all fine too.

The fries are diet wreckers, thanks to their starchy nature but also because of the bad fats in which they're cooked. To improve the taste, some restaurants cook them in beef tallow, which just increases the danger. Even potato chips are a wiser choice. French-fried sweet potatoes are better yet, if cooked in a monounsaturated oil. Best of all: Find another vegetable—like a salad. But if you must have your potatoes once in a while, don't supersize them.

The other lethal member of this trinity, the cola, must of course be replaced with a diet drink at the very least, if you can't go all the way to water.

Replace your typical cheeseburger, fries, and Coke meal with a topless burger (removing the top half of the bun), a salad (such as the McDonald's McSalad Shaker with no cheese and Caesar dressing), and a diet soda, and the carbs drop dramatically.

A Peanut Butter and Jelly Sandwich

The least harmful part of this classic is the peanut butter, of course. It's a good source of monounsaturated fat. It contains resveratrol, too, the same phytochemical that makes red wine beneficial as a protection against heart disease and cancer. Peanut butter also contains folate, which helps you to metabolize homocysteine, a byproduct of protein metabolism that otherwise can harm the cardiovascular system. The drawbacks to commercially processed peanut butter are that bad fats—saturated ones—are sometimes added, and so is sugar. It's best to stick to all-natural peanut butter. Jelly is like eating sugar from the bowl; even teamed with peanut butter, it will jolt your pancreas into making more insulin than is healthy. And the bread you're no doubt using for a base is the standard supermarket white—the worst thing out there. All together, this sandwich is more like a dessert than anything else. Best bet: natural peanut butter with as little jelly as you can stand, on pita or sourdough bread, with skim milk. Even with those modifications, this should be a special treat only.

Pizza and Beer

I'll bet you can guess by now that the oil and the cheese on the pizza aren't the worst things it has to offer. Especially if it's good olive oil and part-skim mozzarella. The crust is white flour, which *is* a problem. And the beer, of course, is nobody's idea of a diet drink. Maltose, the sugar that beer is made from, has a higher glycemic index than white bread. While most of the maltose is fermented out when beer is made, what is left behind are sugars known as "maltodextrins" which also have high glycemic indices. They are probably responsible for an insulin response that leads to the fat storage in the abdomen that we call the beer belly. But pizza isn't completely devoid of benefits. Cooked tomatoes (in the sauce) are a great source of lycopene, a cancer fighter. Completely eliminate pizza and pasta forever and you lose two of the most palatable ways to serve this vegetable. If you can switch from deep dish to thin crust, you've made a difference. And if, along with the olive oil and tomato sauce and part-skim cheese you add some green peppers, onions, mushrooms, and olives, you've added lots of good, nutritious carbs that will make the dish more filling. In place of the beer, try a glass of red wine. Now it's a whole new meal: not quite health food, but better than take-out deep-dish pizza.

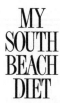

MY SOUTH BEACH DIET

KANDY K.: I NEVER FELT THAT HUNGRY. I read something in the paper about the South Beach Diet just around the time I decided that I needed to lose 15 pounds. And it sounded like a reliable plan—not one of those crazy fad diets you hear about. The fact that it was invented by a cardiologist helped, too. So I started.

Carbs had always been my weakness. I love doughnuts. When you pass a Krispy Kreme place with your son and he wants one, you don't just order one lonely doughnut for him. It's more like: "Well, okay—make that *two* doughnuts." I don't really have a particular problem, but I do like that kind of junk.

The first 2 weeks, the strict phase, were somewhat difficult, because you are so limited. I thought, "You know, this is not going to be as easy as it sounded." Going to restaurants and not having bread was tough. But it was an easy diet, too, because you didn't have to eat certain foods at each meal. You could substitute. If you don't like this, you can have that. If you don't want cheese for a snack, you can have nuts. Which made it very easy to live with. It wasn't prepackaged foods like on some diets where tonight you must have this, and tomorrow for breakfast you have to have this. You can eat the things you like. That was definitely the good part.

And once you grew accustomed to what you could and couldn't have, and you knew the guidelines, then even the strict phase became much easier. I never felt that hungry. You fill up on the things you're allowed to have. So you feel all right. You adjust to it.

I lost about 10 pounds on the diet, but now that I started working with a personal trainer, and I've actually put back about 5 of those pounds in muscle. But I'm much firmer than before—muscle weighs more than fat. There are days when I still want to stop at Krispy Kreme. But now I say, "Oh, no, no—I'm not going to do that again." ∎

IT'S NOT JUST
WHAT YOU EAT,
IT'S HOW
YOU EAT IT

As we've seen, the equation behind most obesity is simple: The faster the sugars and starches you eat are processed and absorbed into your bloodstream, the fatter you get.

Therefore, anything that speeds the process by which your body digests carbohydrates is bad for your diet, and anything that slows it down is good. Digestion is simply the action of your stomach breaking food down into its components; anything that keeps food intact longer is beneficial for people trying to lose weight.

Keeping that in mind, it's important to recognize that the process of digestion begins even before you swallow your food. In fact, it starts the moment you start preparing it. Example: Raw broccoli is crunchy, hard, cold, and covered with a layer of nutritious fiber. If you eat it that way, your stomach has really got to work in order to get at the carbs. That's a good thing. Of course, outside of a cocktail party's crudité table, we almost never eat broccoli raw. First we wash it, then we throw away the toughest part of the stalk, and then we cut it up and boil it or steam it until it's soft and warm.

That's also a fair approximation of what your stomach does to food—through the combination of churning muscles and the potent gastric juices and acids it produces, your stomach physically tears food to shreds and partly liquefies it. Whether it's in a pot on the stove or in your stomach, the same essential process happens to the broccoli and everything else you eat.

In the case of processed foods, digestion begins even earlier—in fact, it starts long before the food hits the supermarket shelf. Consider that loaf of sliced white bread. First the wheat is stripped of the bran and fiber. Then it's pulverized into the finest white flour. The baking process puffs it up into light, airy slices of bread. No wonder your stomach makes such quick work of it. A slice of white bread hits your bloodstream with the same jolt you'd get by eating a tablespoon of table sugar right from the bowl! Marie Antoinette would have a hard time telling it from cake, and the truth is that there's not much difference.

Whereas real, old-fashioned bread—the coarse, chewy kind with a thick crust and visible pieces of grain, the type you can only buy from a bakery or a health food store—puts your stomach to work. It, too, is made of wheat, but the grains haven't been processed to death. You may even see pieces of bran there in the bread. It contains starches, which are just chains of sugars, but they are bound up with the fiber, and so digestion takes longer. As a result, the sugars are released gradually into the bloodstream. If there's no sudden surge in blood sugar, your pancreas won't produce as much insulin, and you won't get the exaggerated craving for more carbs.

This is crucial to understanding how your body operates: The more food is preprocessed, the more fattening it will be.

The good news, of course, is that you can partly control the glycemic index of your food just by choosing how you'll prepare it.

Take a potato, for instance. An incredibly versatile vegetable. You can do a hundred things with it, from soup to vodka. And what you do with it determines how fattening it is.

The worst way, from the glycemic index perspective? Baked. The process of baking it renders the starches most easily accessible to your digestive system.

Slightly better? Believe it or not, that baked potato will be less fattening topped with a dollop of low-fat cheese or sour cream. The calorie count will be slightly higher, but the fat contained in the cheese or sour cream will slow down the digestive process, thereby lessening the amount of insulin that potato prompts your body to make.

(Still, don't think that when you're at the mall and stop for a quick baked potato at one of those franchise places that you're having a healthy snack. A baked potato in midafternoon practically guarantees that you'll be starving for carbs by dinner. You'd be better off having a small ice cream or even a dark chocolate bar instead of that baked potato.)

Better than baked? Mashed or boiled, due to the difference in the cooking process, but also because you'd probably eat them with a little butter or sour cream, and the fat slows the digestive process. Even french fries are better than baked, believe it or not, because of the fat in which they're cooked. Of course, the same is true of potato chips, but don't be misled: None of these are good choices for someone on the South Beach Diet. The type of potato you eat is also a big factor in all this. Red-skinned potatoes are highest in carbs. White-skinned are better. New potatoes, better yet—in every vegetable or fruit, the younger when picked, the lower the carb count. If you must indulge, do so sparingly. And try sweet potatoes instead of white.

The Fiber Factor

How bad is white bread? Worse than ice cream. If you're about to sit down to dinner and need to decide whether to have white bread with it or ice cream after, go for the ice cream—it's less fattening.

But of course, not all bread is white bread. A good rule of thumb is that the coarser and heavier bread is, the better it is for you.

These principles apply across the board: Whole and intact is better than chopped or sliced, which is better than diced, which is better than mashed or pureed—all of which is better than juiced. An apple, for instance, has got a fair amount of pectin, a soluble fiber, in its skin. So if you eat an apple your stomach has got to contend with the fiber before it can get to the fructose. Similarly, an orange has its fiber in the pulp and in the white pithy stuff that clings to the flesh.

But take that apple and peel it, and then juice it, and you've got something quite a bit different. The micronutrients and the fiber are in the skin. With the skin intact, it may take you 5 minutes to eat that apple. But it requires just a few seconds to drink the equivalent in juice. And keep in mind that the glycemic index number is in part determined by the speed with which you eat and digest your food or drink. This is why diabetics having a hypoglycemic reaction quickly drink some orange juice rather than eat the fruit. And while fructose is preferable to sucrose, a big glass of juice acts a lot like a soda—a pure sugar rush. This is especially true of processed juice made without fiber or pulp, which for many people is the only kind they buy.

The fiber delays your stomach's effort to get at the sugars and starches in carbohydrates. The fiber in vegetables like broccoli is cellulose, which is in essence *wood*. The nutrients are bound up in that fiber, too, so the stomach has to work harder to get at the nutrition.

Sugar Stoppers

Fiber's not the only thing that gets in the way of sugars.

Fats and proteins also slow the speed with which your stomach does its job on carbs. Eating a little protein, or some fat—good fat, naturally—along with your carbs is beneficial. A little olive oil on your bread, or some low-fat cheese, is actually better for you than the bread alone. Pasta with tomato sauce and a chunk of Italian bread is an extremely high-carb meal. Such a meal eaten with some meat or cheese is better. Sitting down to a nice baked potato for lunch isn't such a hot idea. Having that potato with a piece of steak and some broccoli renders it better for your diet than a potato on its own. You'll actually make less insulin, and you'll reduce the cravings for more food in the hours ahead.

Here's a tip that will lower the glycemic index of any meal: Fifteen minutes before you begin eating, have a spoonful of Metamucil in a glass of water. It's true, this is normally intended as a mild laxative. But it's simply psyllium, which is fiber—nonsoluble fiber. When you swallow that spoonful, the fiber forms a slippery lump which makes its way through your digestive tract, clearing out anything in its path. When you take some before eating, the fiber gets mixed in with the food and has the effect of slowing the speed with which your stomach digests what you've eaten.

When we talk about diet we talk so exclusively about the things we eat that it's easy to forget how much has to do with the things we drink. But your body doesn't make that distinction—by the time your meal reaches your small intestine, it's *all* liquid.

In fact, what you drink is critical because it requires little digestion and therefore goes more directly into your bloodstream. If there's sugar in that beverage, it will speed into your system, prompting the burst of insulin that leads to cravings later on.

At one end of the drink spectrum, to no one's surprise, is water. By now we've all heard the health gospel that we need at least 2 or 3 quarts of it a day. There's some question about whether we really require *quite* so much, but a good rule is to reach for water whenever you're thirsty. It's especially good for dieters because it creates the sensation of a full belly.

At the other end of the spectrum is beer. As discussed, its major carbohydrate components called maltodextrins have glycemic indices that are higher than table sugar.

Wine, and even whiskey, are safer bets because they're made from different grains, vegetables, or fruit. Not that whiskey is part of any serious weight-loss effort, of course. White wine is better. Best of all is red wine, because it brings with it some significant, proven cardiac benefits thanks to the resveratrol contained in the grape skins.

It's no surprise that sodas are a major source of sugar, so I won't belabor it. Sweetened iced teas aren't much better.

Coffee, of course, contains no sugar on its own. People have grown accustomed to hearing doctors advise against excesses, but I don't think they're all that bad in moderation. Some diets steer people toward decaf for the simple reason that caffeine does stimulate the pancreas to produce insulin, which is the last thing an overweight person needs. Still, the effect isn't all that great, and if a cup or two of coffee a day makes you happy, I think you should feel free. Tea may actually play a role in the prevention of heart attack and prostate cancer.

Again, fruit juices are a big source of trouble, in part because we've come to associate them with healthy habits. They do carry nutrients, especially freshly made juices. But they also bring with them high levels of fructose, which can be the undoing of any effort to lose weight.

Because I live in Florida, the best fruit example I can think of is the orange. A patient of mine began experiencing symptoms of diabetes. His blood sugar was suddenly up over 400, not a good sign. He didn't have any of the conditions that usually are present with new onset diabetes, such as an infection or other stress on his system. I began quizzing him about any changes to his eating habits when he mentioned that a juice machine had just been installed in his office. He thought he was making a healthy choice by having several glasses of orange juice a day to replace the coffee he once favored.

Cut the juice, I advised him—you're dumping too much sugar into your bloodstream. He switched to water and his blood sugar returned to normal.

Therein lies everything you need to know about fruit juice. If you were to eat an orange you'd get the same fructose as in the juice. But you'd also be getting a lot of fiber in the flesh and pulp and membranes. Your stomach would have to work to separate the sugar from everything else in the course of digestion. In addition, you might eat one orange at a sitting, maybe two if you were hungry or if they were on the small side. But peeling an orange is work, and eating one takes time.

Not surprisingly, store-bought juice is the worst offender.

Fresh-squeezed, because of the fibrous pulp and the superior nutrients, is better.

This holds for nearly all fruit juices. Pineapple juice? Just loaded with sugar. Grape? The same. All of a sudden, it seems, America's parents fell in love with apple juice and began giving it to their kids with every meal. From a sugar consumption point of view, this was a bad idea. The skin of an apple is actually quite healthy—the pectin is a good fiber that accompanies the fructose into your system. So eating an apple a day is still a prescription for well-being. But drinking its juice is not.

If you must have fruit juice, try just a splash of it in sparkling water—a spritzer, in other words.

When it comes to vegetable juices you've got a bit more latitude. But the health food store mainstay—fresh carrot juice—isn't on the approved list. As we've noted elsewhere, carrots have a high glycemic index. Beet juice is said to be good for many reasons, but it, too, is loaded with sugars. I've heard that tossing a banana into the blender along with a little milk and some berries, accompanied by ice, makes a good summer smoothie. But bananas are among the worst fruits in terms of fructose content. If you knew nothing about nutrition and were asked to guess which fruits and vegetables contain the most sugar, you'd probably fare pretty well. The sweeter the taste, the more sugar is present. Watermelon is bad. Tomatoes are better. Broccoli juice would be best, if anybody actually wanted to indulge in a glass every day with breakfast. So be glad that the South Beach Diet doesn't require a big glass of broccoli juice every day.

MY SOUTH BEACH DIET

KATIE A.: I NEVER FEEL LIKE I'M MISSING A THING.

I've watched my weight since I was about 7 years old. That's when my sister and I spent a summer visiting my grandmother in Pennsylvania, and we ate all the processed and packaged foods she had in the house—and she didn't cook. She owned a business, and to keep us busy she'd give us money so we'd scoot down to the candy shop. My sister and I came back home from that summer looking like roly-polies.

I've been battling my weight ever since. You name the diet, I've been on it. I even found a doctor who gave me injections to perk up my thyroid gland so I'd lose weight. I ended up with Graves' disease. I was on Weight Watchers, too. And, yes, I did lose the weight, and I got the pin and all that jazz. But you know what happens? You become so obsessed with food, and you're thinking so much in terms of categorizing your food—I mean: How many breads? How many fruits? How many this or that? You find that you're thinking about food 24-7!

My hang-up was carbs and sweets. I was working the evening shift at the hospital back then, so I didn't get to bed till 4 A.M.. I'd start eating while still on the floor because the patients were always getting cookies and candies. When you got a little tired, you saw everybody else sitting around snacking. You weren't necessarily hungry, just tired, so you went for the food. Then, I'd get home and I'd feel guilty about all the junk I ate at work. I'd say: Well, now you've got to eat something healthy. So I'd have dinner, and *then* I'd go to bed. All my eating was done between 3 in the afternoon and maybe 3 in the morning. I'd get up for work and only have coffee for breakfast—and come to work on the 3-to-11 shift. I knew that you weren't supposed to eat after 8 o'clock at night. But that shift puts you on an abnormal clock. It was chips, and pretzels, and all of that. Banana chips *and* sweets—and cookies and cake. Bread. Rice. That was it. And in my mind I said: Well, I'm not eating *that* much. Because I was piecemealing. A little at a time. I was also a tremendous caffeine drinker back then. I was drinking a six-pack of soda every day—Diet Coke, or Diet Pepsi, or Tab. But it definitely was not caffeine-free, and I learned later that the caffeine was an appetite stimulant for me.

I didn't gain it all at once—the pounds just started to creep on. Until one day, my mother was walking behind me at the mall, and she caught up and said, "You know something? You're starting to *waddle*."

That did it. That was 2 years ago, when I went on this diet. I lost 30 pounds since then, and I've kept it off. The best thing about this diet is that it is easy to stick to. It's even flexible. For instance: I cheated almost from day one. Maybe not during the first 2 weeks, the strict phase. But after that. You could have nuts, let's say, but you were supposed to count out just 30 of them as a portion. Well, some nights I didn't count.

But beyond that, I've stuck with it, unlike all those other diets I tried. I haven't had a piece of bread in 2 years. Not a grain of rice, either. It's a self-control issue. But at the same time, I don't feel as though I'm denying myself. There's plenty that I can eat on this diet. And I have lots of positive results that keep me going. I know now that I can go into a store and I won't be reaching for that size 16. I'm now between a 10 and a 12, and I'm comfortable with that.

I've been able to stick to this diet so well that about a year ago I confessed to the nutritionist at Mount Sinai that I hadn't had an apple or any other fruit in over a year. And she got all over my case. "Katie, you should know better," she said. Anyway, I'm eating every kind of fruit now. Lots of vegetables, lots of fruits, lots of salads. But I know a lot more about what I eat than I did before. Like, people don't realize that the MSG in their Chinese food is made from beets, which contain a *lot* of sugar. Or that carrots have a high glycemic index, too. I used to eat a lot of carrots, especially when I was trying to lose weight. I even traveled with little bags of them. So I was shocked to learn that carrots have so much sugar in them. You don't realize that those carrots, or those onions, just turn right into sugar that gets stored in your body as fat.

Lately I actually gained a few pounds back—I'll be honest with you—because I cheated with those nuts. I'm into cashews now, but I've done the whole gamut. I've done peanuts. And almonds. Again, you don't realize that there's sugar in nuts, too. Pistachios are wonderful on this diet, because you can have only 15 almonds but 30 pistachio nuts, because they're so small. And I think I've begun to overdo it with the pistachios, and I may have put a few pounds back on. But I don't even get on the scale anymore. I go by how I feel in my clothing. Because I don't want to do a number on my head with weighing myself every day. If I feel like I'm getting too carried away with the nuts, I back off. And I drop a few pounds. Just recently I found a baker who makes sugar-free cheesecake. I buy it and cut it into very small portions. Then, when I get a yen for it—it's not every night, it might be two or three times a week—I'll just go ahead and take a piece and defrost it. It's something that I can have. It's enough. And so I never feel like I'm missing a thing. ■

HOW EATING
MAKES YOU
HUNGRY

How eating makes you *what*?

Weren't you always under the impression that eating is what *satisfies* hunger?

Well, it is and it isn't. Eating does put an immediate end to hunger. But some foods also create new cravings by making you hungrier than you would be if you hadn't eaten them.

This isn't just a theory, or a matter of perception.

Dr. David S. Ludwig is the head of the obesity program at Children's Hospital in Boston, a physician who also teaches at Harvard Medical School. Dr. Ludwig recently studied how the breakfast eaten by some obese teenagers influenced their hunger levels hours later.

Three groups of overweight adolescents were fed breakfasts of identical calorie counts. One group's meal was 20 percent fat, 16 percent protein, and roughly two-thirds carbs, but the good kind—steel-cut oatmeal, meaning the flakes were large and the kernel of the oat was unprocessed, and so the fiber was intact. The second group also had a two-thirds-carbs breakfast, but they were served *instant* oatmeal, where the fiber has been stripped away to permit shorter cooking time.

The third group's meal was identical to a typical South Beach Diet breakfast—vegetable omelets.

After breakfast, members of all three groups were instructed to eat anything they wanted for the next 5 hours.

The subjects who had the bad carb breakfast—the instant oatmeal group—ate the most during that 5-hour period. They also reported feeling the strongest hunger pangs.

The teenagers who had the steel-cut oatmeal felt less hunger and ate less than the instant oatmeal group during the postbreakfast hours.

The group who had the vegetable omelets—the low-carb meal—reported the lowest sensation of hunger and ate the smallest amount during the 5 hours after breakfast.

This is one of several recent studies testing the theory that eating bad carbs makes you hungrier, and that on a diet of good carbs and good fats (the vegetable omelet combines both) you'll want less food later. I'll explain exactly why this happens, but for now I want to emphasize what all the studies show: Eating bad carbohydrates—especially highly processed ones—creates cravings for more bad carbs, which ultimately is responsible for our epidemic of obesity. It's hard to overstate the connection between bad carbs, obesity, and bad cardiac health.

In another diet and hunger study, subjects who ate whole fruit reported less hunger than those who ate puree of the same fruit, and those who ate puree had fewer cravings than those who just drank the juice. In various other research projects, scientists found that eating beans causes less hunger than eating potatoes; raw carrots cause less hunger than cooked ones; foods containing whole grains cause less hunger than those containing cracked grains; ordinary rice causes less hunger than the instant variety.

There's a term for the basic physiological response to food that's behind all these findings: reactive hypoglycemia.

I will describe exactly what that means. But before I tell you, let me show you.

For years, every day at around 3 or 4 in the afternoon, I'd find myself running out of steam—weak, sleepy, sometimes even light-headed. Without thinking, I'd make a run for the doctors' lounge, where I would inhale a bran muffin and a cup of coffee. I actually thought that since the muffin was labeled low fat, it was healthy. In fact, the word *bran* was there mainly to keep people from examining the ingredients closely and realizing that the muffin was just a cupcake in disguise. I was lulled into a false sense of security—the fat in the muffin may have been low, but the carbs it contained contributed quite a bit of fat to my waistline.

Having finished my snack, I instantly felt better. So give my body credit for knowing exactly what it needed: Carbs. *Sugar.* My body knew this because it detected that the level of glucose—the form sugar takes in our bloodstreams—had fallen too low. Glucose is a form of chemical energy that our brains in particular need on a constant basis in order to function properly. Without enough, we'd grow dizzy, faint, and eventually go into a coma and die. Diabetes is the body's inability to turn food into usable forms of energy; this is why without synthetic insulin, type 1 diabetics would not live for long.

So my brain detects hypoglycemia—too-low blood sugar—and my body reacts (hence the name reactive hypoglycemia) by creating the cravings that drove me, and maybe you, too, toward the nearest carbohydrate fix.

How Carbs Work

As we've already said, carbohydrates are contained in a vast and varied array of foods, everything from the most virtuous vegetable to the most decadent treat. All carbs contain sugars. These sugars, though, exist in several different forms and go by a variety of names, including maltose (in beer), sucrose (table sugar), lactose (in dairy), and fructose (as found in fruit).

Despite that similarity, no one who has ever craved a sugar doughnut has been satisfied by broccoli. The opposite might also be true, though it's difficult to find people who suffer from insatiable cravings for green vegetables.

It's easy to tell by taste which carbs are highest in sugars, and which yield their sugars most readily. It probably comes as no surprise that a milk chocolate bar gives up its sugars more freely than one made of dark chocolate, or a pineapple yields its sweetness faster than a grapefruit, or a slice of supermarket white bread produces blood sugar faster than a coarse-grained health food cracker. The more sugar there is, and the faster it's released, the more acutely we sense that sugar "rush"—the relief that courses through our bloodstream as we heed the call for carbs. Internally, though, our bodies treat all carbs in basically the same way—digestion is in large part the process by which our bodies extract the sugars from carbohydrates and turn them into fuel, which we either burn or store. Burning the fuel is good—that means we're active enough to make efficient use of the food we eat. Storage of a little fuel is all right, but anything more than that is not so good. You know that excess stored fuel by another term: body fat.

The job of carbohydrate digestion starts in our mouths, when we chew the food into bits and our saliva begins the chemical process of separating each mouthful into its components. In our stomachs, the food is further shredded by the organ's muscular contractions and gastric acids. Our bodies want to get at the sugars contained in carbs, but this happens at varying speeds, depending on certain factors. Essentially, the less encumbered these sugars are by other substances, the faster they enter our bloodstreams.

Carbs' Competitors

Which substances get in our bodies' way? Fiber is the major factor that slows the absorption of sugar. That's the reason the highly processed oatmeal was worse, diet-wise, than the steel-cut variety—the latter had all the fiber still intact, and so before the stomach could get to the sugars in the oatmeal, it had to separate them from the fiber. Once isolated, the fiber passes undigested through your system; its dietary importance comes from its ability to slow digestion down. It's an obstacle to digestion—a good one.

This was proven not long ago in a scientific study in which half the subjects were given the fiber known as psyllium (you probably know it better as Metamucil) 15 minutes before lunch. The other half had lunch without the psyllium first. In the hours after the meal, the fiber group reported less hunger than the others. As the day wore on they ate less, too. The reason is simple: In their stomachs, the psyllium mixed in with what they ate and drank and slowed down the digestion. Slower digestion of carbs, less insulin. Less insulin, less dramatic drop in blood sugar. Less of a sugar rise and fall now, less hunger later.

Fiber isn't the only thing that slows the digestion of carbohydrates. Fat, too, slows the speed at which your small intestine accesses the sugars you've eaten. That's why, in the study of overweight adolescents, the omelet breakfast created the least desire to eat more later. We have found other factors that slow the digestion of carbs and therefore benefit dieters. Acidic foods such as lemon and vinegar slow the speed with which your stomach empties, therefore cutting back on the rise in blood sugar. You can dress salads or vegetables in both and enjoy the benefit. Even sourdough bread, while not high in fiber, is acidic, and will slow stomach emptying and thereby slow digestion.

This is an important lesson in eating properly and losing weight on the South Beach Diet. This is why we call carbs containing fiber *good*, and why we also think of certain fats as good, too: Anything that slows the process by which you process the sugars in carbs is by definition, good.

The Body's Response

Once the food has been liquefied in the stomach, it travels downward to our small intestines, where millions of capillaries absorb what we've eaten and transport it into our bloodstreams. Once there, it travels through our livers and then everywhere else in our bodies to be used, stored, or eliminated.

But let's continue to focus on the carbs. As we've said, they all contain sugar in one form or another. Even the starches are merely chains of sugars; digestion cuts the links in order to make the sugar molecules available to us. What we're concerned with here is the *speed* with which our bodies get at the sugars. It doesn't all take place at the same rate.

Once the sugars enter our bloodstreams, it is the job of the pancreas to detect this and go to work—producing the hormone insulin in sufficient quantity to get the sugars out of our blood and into the organs where it is needed, or into storage for future needs. This is where diabetics run into trouble: They ingest the same sugars as everyone else, but without effective insulin those sugars remain uselessly circulating in the bloodstream. Insulin unlocks our tissues and lets the sugars in.

Fortunately, the pancreas can tell how much insulin is needed to do that job. If the body experiences a fast infusion of sugars, a lot of insulin is required. If the sugars are metabolized more slowly, the insulin is released gradually.

This is a crucial difference, as far as obesity is concerned: Fast sugar is worse for you; slower is better.

Here's why. When the sugars are absorbed slowly, the rise in blood sugar is gradual, and so is its descent once the insulin begins to do its work. The slow decline in blood sugar translates into less insistent cravings for more carbs later. You recall what I described as reactive hypoglycemia—the sensation of hunger caused by low blood sugar. When the decline in blood sugar is gentle, the cravings are lessened.

But when your pancreas detects a rapid rise in blood sugar, it pumps out a correspondingly high level of insulin to do the job. That results in a rapid plunge in the blood sugar level. The insulin ends up doing its job a little too well—the blood sugar level drops so low that new cravings are created, requiring more quick carbohydrate fixes. In order to satisfy so many cravings, of course, we take in well beyond the nutrition we require. We overeat, and this leads to more fat, more insulin resistance, more hunger, and more weight gain—a vicious cycle.

Therefore, we can most easily stop ourselves from overeating by two strategies:

1. We can eat the foods (and combinations of foods) that cause gradual rather than sharp increases and decreases in blood sugar.

2. We can learn to anticipate hypoglycemia and avert it with the timely consumption of snacks. This one is crucial: It takes much less food to prevent hypoglycemia than it does to resolve it.

The third thing we all should do is learn which foods cause the most rapid rise in blood sugar. In the early 1980s, Dr. David Jenkins led a team of Canadian researchers who devised a scale to measure the rapidity and degree with which a fixed quantity of a food increases your blood sugar. They called it the glycemic index. It lists most carbohydrates, from table sugar, beer, and white bread at one extreme to spinach and lentils at the other. On page 70 you will find a sample of the index, organized by food type. You probably won't be completely surprised by what you find there. Anything made with white flour is high on the list. That includes most desserts, breads, and baked goods, of course, but also pasta. Instant rice is also near the top. Certain tropical fruits are fairly high, as are some starchy vegetables, particularly potatoes and other root vegetables. The king of all sugars, the one that increases blood sugar faster than any other, is maltose, which exists in beer (but is largely removed when beer is brewed). However, the sugar molecules called maltodextrins remain and have a similar effect on blood sugar. Now you understand what's behind the beer belly: The rapid rise of blood sugar caused by guzzling this beverage stimulates a corresponding rise in insulin production, which encourages storage of fat around the midsection.

Knowledge and use of the glycemic index of foods is becoming widespread, but there's an important caveat that is crucial to understanding the link between carbs and obesity. You must bear in mind that the degree to which your blood sugar is raised depends not just on the glycemic index of the food but also on the quantity. For example, carrots have a high glycemic index, but they are fairly low in carbohydrate density. Therefore, you'd have to eat several handfuls of carrots to approximate the total rise in blood sugar you'd get from a single slice of white bread.

I have a handy analogy I use to explain this concept to my patients.

Think of alcohol. When we drink it, our blood alcohol level rises, and when it goes above a certain threshold, we feel tipsy. When it rises further, we feel drunk. We know that when we drink on an empty stomach, we get drunk faster. If, on the other hand we drink while eating, and have a full stomach, it takes more alcohol for us to feel the effect. This is because when the drinks mix with the food in our stomach, it delays the absorption of the alcohol into our bloodstream. Once in the bloodstream, it's transported to our brain, creating that intoxicated sensation. The principle at work here is this: The more slowly the alcohol is absorbed, the less it affects us.

Now let's consider what happens when we eat carbs—bread, for instance.

If we eat white bread, we're getting no fiber with our carbs. That's like drinking on an empty stomach: Our stomachs can get at the starches without having to first separate them from the fiber. As a result, the bread is quickly turned into glucose—blood sugar—and causes an equally sharp rise in insulin, which brings about the dreaded acute rise and fall of blood sugar level, creating more cravings later on. Eating white bread is analogous to drinking alcohol on an empty stomach; eating whole grain bread is like eating with your cocktail.

The fiber is the part of the grain not absorbed into the bloodstream from the intestine but excreted as waste. Even though it is not absorbed, fiber helps digestion in another, more commonly understood way. It helps your colon to function efficiently. The lack of fiber in our diets is one reason why constipation has become a common problem.

Fiber, then, joins fat, protein, and acidity on the list of things that delay the absorption of sugars and starches. We need to include one or more of the above in every meal in order to keep ourselves from getting drunk— on carbs. By choosing the right foods, food combinations, and strategically timed snacks, you can prevent hypoglycemia and thereby control your weight without having to fight off cravings.

A final anecdote to illustrate this principle: A friend and patient who was in the first week of the diet rushed out one afternoon to play golf. He had neglected to plan his lunch so he decided to break the rules and grab a sandwich. As he played golf, several hours later, he began to feel weak and shaky and recognized this as reactive hypoglycemia. There were no permissible snacks available, so he found some sugar packets and guzzled them down. They relieved his acute hunger and they tasted great, too. He returned home and downed a bag of tortilla chips and a chocolate bar. This binge was due not to a loss of self-control but to his poor planning. Once the hypoglycemia struck, the consequence was preordained. Had my friend eaten tuna salad instead of a sandwich and had some low-fat cheese or nuts as a snack, both the initial hypoglycemia and subsequent gorging could have been avoided.

MY SOUTH BEACH DIET

PAUL L.: I'VE CLEANED OUT MY MEDICINE CABINET THANKS TO THIS DIET. I weighed 232 pounds 5 years ago, when I went on this diet. Over the years, I had always struggled with my weight, and I tried lots of the diets out there. I tried Atkins—in fact, I had actually been a patient of his years ago, before he got famous. And so I tried his low-carb diet. I also tried some of the low-fat diets, the Heart Association-type programs. I always lost some weight, but I always gained it back.

I'm 73 now, and I was 68 when I started with the South Beach Diet.

I had been a heavy smoker and then I gave it up, which is how I happened to put on all that weight. I wasn't a big sweets eater. But I loved all the rest. Bread three times a day, with every meal. And potatoes. Rice. Pasta. Of course, meat and so on—big, heavy meals. Once my weight hit its peak, I started getting some other problems, too. One day we found that I had diabetes. My blood pressure was high. My triglycerides were high. My cholesterol was high.

I began seeing Dr. Agatston as my cardiologist, and we discussed how my being so overweight was contributing to my conditions. He suggested the diet he developed. And because I was no stranger to diets, I said I'd give it a try.

The first few days weren't exactly easy. I wouldn't say you feel bad, but definitely different. A little off. You're hungry because you're not following your normal eating patterns. But after those first 3 days, it suddenly seemed easier. I wasn't really going hungry. I ate a ton of vegetables during that strict phase, and a lot of meat and fish and cheese, too. A lot of white meat chicken and turkey. But no bread or pasta or even fruit.

After the first 2 weeks, I started adding things back into my diet. I had some fruit, although to be honest, when I had a little fruit I wanted more. It was easier in a way to just go without fruit altogether.

I never did add any potatoes back to my diet—I just didn't miss them enough to want them, I guess. And maybe it's easier for me to have none than a little. I do like pasta, and so I'll have that every once in a while—say, every few weeks I'll have a dish. Rice, less so, though I'll have that occasionally, too. I have gone back to eating bread. I'll have it just about every day now, and two or three pieces. And I drink red wine—two glasses a day.

It took me about a year, but I went from 232 down to 170 on this diet. Sixty pounds in 50 weeks. And for the past 4 years I've been maintaining this weight pretty easily. Once it crept up again, to 178, so I just went back on the Phase 1 diet and I got back down to 170 pretty fast.

The best part, though, is that I've cleaned out my medicine cabinet thanks to this diet. I stopped taking the diabetes medicine because it cleared up. Blood pressure medicine—gone. I was taking a statin for my cholesterol, but now I've even thrown that away. ∎

THE GLYCEMIC INDEX

The following table lists the glycemic index of many of the foods you're likely to encounter in your daily life. The choices are grouped by type of food, then arranged in each group from foods with the lowest glycemic index to those with the highest.

A food's glycemic index is the amount that it increases your blood sugar compared to the amount that the same quantity of white bread would increase it.

The foods with the lower numbers will cause your blood sugar to rise then fall more slowly than the foods with higher numbers will. Numerous studies have also shown that low-glycemic foods satisfy your hunger longer and minimize your food cravings better.

In Phase 1 of the South Beach Diet, you should only choose foods with a low glycemic index. Later on, after you've gone through the rapid weight-loss phase, you can start mixing in foods with higher numbers.

However, still follow the other rules of the diet; even though low-fat milk and peanut M&Ms have the same glycemic index, the milk is a much better nutritional choice.

BAKERY PRODUCTS	GI
Sponge cake	66
Pound cake	77
Danish	84
Muffin	88
Flan	93
Angel food cake	95
Croissant	96
Doughnut	108
Waffles	109

BEVERAGES	GI
Soy milk	43

	GI
Apple juice (unsweetened)	57
Pineapple juice	66
Grapefruit juice	69

BREADS	GI
Oat bran bread	68
Mixed grain bread	69
Pumpernickel	71
White pita	82
Cheese pizza	86
Hamburger bun	87
Rye flour bread	92
Semolina bread	92

Oat kernel bread	93
Whole wheat bread	99
Melba toast	100
White bread	101
Plain Bagel	103
Kaiser rolls	104
Bread stuffing	106
Gluten-free wheat bread	129
French baguette	136

BREAKFAST CEREALS	GI
Rice bran	27
All-Bran	60
Oatmeal, noninstant	70
Special K	77
Kellogg's Smacks	78
Oat bran	78
Muesli	80
Kellogg's Mini-Wheats (whole wheat)	81
Bran Chex	83
Kellogg's Just Right	84
Life	94
Grape-Nuts	96
Shredded Wheat	99
Cream of Wheat	100
Golden Grahams	102
Puffed Wheat	105
Cheerios	106
Corn Bran	107
Total	109
Rice Krispies	117
Corn Chex	118

Cornflakes	119
Crispix	124
Rice Chex	127

CEREAL GRAINS	GI
Pearled barley	36
Rye	48
Wheat kernels	59
Rice, instant	65
Bulgur	68
Rice, parboiled	68
Cracked barley	72
Wheat, quick cooking	77
Buckwheat	78
Brown rice	79
Wild rice	81
White rice	83
Couscous	93
Rolled barley	94
Mahatma Premium Rice	94
Taco shells	97
Cornmeal	98
Millet	101
Tapioca, boiled with milk	115

COOKIES	GI
Oatmeal cookies	79
Shortbread	91
Arrowroot	95
Graham crackers	106
Vanilla wafers	110
Biscotti	113

CRACKERS	GI
Breton wheat crackers	96
Stoned wheat thins	96
Rice cakes	110

DAIRY FOODS	GI
Low fat yogurt, artifically sweetened	20
Chocolate milk, artifically sweetened	34
Whole milk	39
Fat-free milk	46
Low fat yogurt, fruit flavored	47
Low-fat ice cream	71
Ice cream	87

FRUIT AND FRUIT PRODUCTS	GI
Cherries	32
Apple	34
Grapefruit	36
Peach	40
Dried apricots	43
Fresh apricots	43
Canned peach	43
Orange	47
Pear	47
Plum	55
Apple juice	56
Grapes	62
Canned pear	63
Raisins	64
Pineapple juice	66
Grapefruit juice	69
Fruit cocktail	79
Kiwifruit	83
Mango	86
Banana	89
Canned apricots, in syrup	91
Pineapple	94
Watermelon	103

LEGUMES	GI
Soybeans, boiled	23
Red lentils, boiled	36
Kidney beans, boiled	42
Green lentils, boiled	42
Butter beans, boiled	44
Yellow split peas, boiled	45
Baby lima beans, frozen	46
Chickpeas	47
Navy beans, boiled	54
Pinto beans	55
Black-eyed peas	59
Canned chickpeas	60
Canned pinto beans	64
Canned baked beans	69
Canned kidney beans	74
Canned green lentils	74
Fava beans	113

PASTA	GI
Protein-enriched spaghetti	38
Fettuccine	46
Vermicelli	50

Whole grain spaghetti	53
Meat-filled ravioli	56
White spaghetti	59
Capellini	64
Macaroni	64
Linguine	65
Cheese tortellini	71
Durum spaghetti	78
Macaroni and cheese	92
Gnocchi	95
Brown rice pasta	113

ROOT VEGETABLES	GI
Sweet potato	63
Carrots, cooked	70
Yam	73
White potato, boiled	83
Potato, steamed	93
Potato, mashed	100
New potato	101
Rutabaga	103
Potato, boiled, mashed	104
French fries	107
Potato, instant	114
Potato, microwaved	117
Parsnips	139
Potato, baked	158

SNACK FOOD AND CANDY	GI
Peanuts	21
Mars M&Ms (peanut)	46

Mars Snickers Bar	57
Mars Twix Cookie Bars (caramel)	62
Chocolate bar, 1.5 oz	70
Jams and marmalades	70
Potato chips	77
Popcorn	79
Mars Kudos Whole Grain Bars (chocolate chip)	87
Mars Bar	91
Mars Skittles	98
Life Savers	100
Corn chips	105
Jelly beans	114
Pretzels	116
Dates	146

SOUPS	GI
Canned tomato soup	54
Canned Lentil soup	63
Split pea soup	86
Black bean soup	92
Canned green pea soup	94

SUGARS	GI
Fructose	32
Lactose	65
Honey	83
High-fructose corn syrup	89
Sucrose	92
Glucose	137
Maltodextrin	150
Maltose	150

VEGETABLES	GI
Artichoke	<20
Arugula	<20
Asparagus	<20
Broccoli	<20
Brussels sprouts	<20
Cabbage, all varieties	<20
Cauliflower	<20
Celery	<20
Cucumbers	<20
Escarole	<20
Eggplant	<20
Beet	<20
Chard	<20
Collard	<20
Kale	<20
Mustard	<20
Spinach	<20

Turnip	<20
Lettuce, all varieties	<20
Mushrooms, all varieties	<20
Okra	<20
Peanuts	<20
Peppers, all varieties	<20
Green beans	<20
Snow peas	<20
Spaghetti squash	<20
Young summer squash	<20
Watercress	<20
Wax beans	<20
Zucchini	<20
Tomatoes	23
Dried peas	32
Green peas	68
Sweet corn	78
Pumpkin	107

IS IT DIABETES YET?

I see an awful lot of people with the condition largely responsible for the current epidemic of obesity and heart disease. You see them, too, whether you know it or not.

I see them in my examining room, of course, but I also see them on the street, at parties, at the mall, on the beach, virtually everywhere I look. They're very easy to recognize thanks to one unmistakable visible sign: central obesity—excess weight concentrated mainly in a rounded, protruding waistline, often on individuals with the face, arms, and legs you'd expect to find on someone thinner. It's commonly referred to as apple-shaped obesity—as opposed to pear-shaped, where the excess weight is distributed throughout the hips, buttocks, and legs.

People usually refer to central obesity by some cute euphemism—it's a paunch, a beer gut, a potbelly. But to me it's a serious warning of unhealthy blood chemistry today and cardiac trouble ahead. In social settings, I have to restrain myself from urging people I've just met who fit the above profile to call me (or any cardiologist) first thing in the morning to schedule diagnostic blood tests. I've become something of an evangelist on this subject because the disorder is so widespread and dangerous, yet simple to treat using diet, exercise, and medication.

When I ask overweight patients about family medical history, they'll frequently tell me about a parent or grandparent who developed diabetes late in life, often in their seventies or eighties. "But it was just 'chemical' diabetes," the patient will assure me, using an outdated term. "He didn't even take insulin for it." Sometimes they'll refer to it as "sugar" diabetes, another relic of medical terminology. The patient has no idea that this late-occurring form of the disease in a parent is actually an indication that another, silent but potentially deadly condition is present—one that is setting the stage, internally, for his or her own future heart attack or stroke. The diabetes gene is passed along to all offspring. An early manifestation of the disease is weight gain during middle age—years before blood sugar becomes elevated.

But what does diabetes have to do with a heart attack or stroke? That's the question most people ask. Over the past 10 years we have come a long way in understanding the connection. We now know without a doubt that they are linked: About half of all people who have heart attacks are found to be suffering from a condition that goes under several names. Metabolic syndrome is the most popular current term, but it's also been called insulin resistance, or syndrome X. We've known of its existence only since 1989, and we're still learning about it. For our purposes let's refer to it as prediabetes, since that comes closest to calling it what it is—an early stage of the disease. Unchecked, prediabetes today will turn into full-blown type 2 diabetes tomorrow.

By the latest count, somewhere around 47 million Americans—close to one in five—are estimated to have prediabetes. But the percentage of adults with cardiovascular disease who also have this syndrome is much higher; maybe half of my practice shows signs. Here's a list of the criteria, according the National Cholesterol Education Program.

- High cholesterol
- High ratio of bad cholesterol to good
- High blood pressure
- Central obesity
- High triglycerides

To which I would add:

• Small LDL (bad cholesterol) particles

These are also the conditions that are closely associated with heart attack and stroke. Genetics plays a major role in determining whether you'll have these conditions. But so does improper diet. I'll try not to burden you with too much science as I explain the connection between heart disease and adult-onset diabetes. Trust me: It's important to understand this.

The Facts on Diabetes

Most people know diabetes as the body's inability to process sugars and starches properly. Your body digests a meal and converts all the carbs into glucose—blood sugar. It then becomes the job of your pancreas to detect this sudden infusion of glucose and, in response, produce the hormone insulin. The insulin is needed to allow your body's various organs—brain, muscles, liver, and so on—to extract the glucose from your bloodstream and either use it at once or store it for future use. The body's need for sugar is constant—without it in sufficient quantities you will become dizzy, faint, go into a coma, and before long, die.

Imagine that each cell in your body has a lock on it, and insulin is the only key that fits. If the cells remain locked, the sugars can't enter, and they remain circulating uselessly in your bloodstream, where they do you no good and cause considerable harm.

But what most people don't realize is that diabetes isn't just about how we process sugars: it's also the inability to properly process the fats we eat.

When we eat fats, whether from flesh, vegetable oils, or dairy products, it is also insulin's job to transport the fatty acids (the basic component of fats) from the bloodstream into the body's tissues, where they belong, to be used immediately for fuel or stored for future use in the form we know as triglycerides or simply as fat.

In fact, diabetes can be seen as the body's inability to manage its fuel supply well. Obesity, too, is just a matter of bad fuel management, due to a combination of genetics and lifestyle. Our bodies are designed to store excess energy (which we call calories) for a very good reason. For most of humanity's existence, securing a steady and sufficient supply of food has been our biggest, most important challenge. Feast or famine prevailed, and to adapt, our bodies would save the energy from today's feast, knowing that tomorrow it would need to burn saved fuel in order to survive. That's why this particular brand of obesity concentrates the fat in the midsection—it leaves the extremities lithe and muscular, for ease of manual labor and, especially, flight. Advanced civilization has done a great deal to eradicate famine, but at the expense of our waistlines and our cardiovascular systems, which now suffer from stored fat that we no longer need. We would be better off if our bodies eliminated excess energy as if it were waste, but they don't.

This is exacerbated by the physiology of the fat cell. When we gain weight, we're not creating new fat cells—their number remains constant from childhood. No, what happens is that the fat cells themselves get fat. That's why in overweight people the insulin has trouble attaching to the fat cells—they've grown too big. As a result, when an overweight person overeats, it's like trying to fill a gas tank that's already at capacity—the excess spills over. In your body, that means the sugars and fats circulate in your blood longer than they should. When your body cannot properly transfer the glucose and fatty acids from your bloodstream into your tissues, it's the beginning of trouble. Left untreated, serious cases of diabetes are fatal.

But there are *two* types of diabetes, and these differ in important ways.

Juvenile (or type 1) diabetes usually strikes during childhood or adolescence. It's caused by some damage that's been done to the pancreas—possibly by a virus. As a result, the organ produces too little insulin to do the job of getting sugars and fats from the bloodstream into the proper tissues. It's an incurable disease at this point and can be treated only by replacing the insulin with daily insulin injections. That's why eating carefully and measuring blood sugar level are so important to a diabetic's well-being and why insulin is such a lifesaving drug.

We don't even have a proper name yet for the other form of this disease; hence its working title: type 2 diabetes. This is also called adult-onset diabetes, because that's when it usually shows up. As we've said, there's no virus to blame, just who we are (genetics) and what we eat. A surprisingly large percentage of us are genetically predisposed to diabetes of this kind. But the predisposition is just that—the *potential* for diabetes—until poor diet and lack of exercise do their damage. We can't control our genes. But if you can keep from making bad food choices, you can prevent this form of diabetes.

Both these diseases go by the same name, but the causes are opposite. Juvenile diabetes is a result of the pancreas's inability to produce insulin. In type 2, your pancreas is fully functional and is actually making *too much* insulin. When you carry excess body fat, you make it difficult for insulin to do its job. So the blood sugar level doesn't drop as quickly as it should, prompting your pancreas to pump out even more insulin in order to unlock your cells and let the glucose in. Your pancreas sends out insulin until finally it overshoots the mark, which is why the blood sugar level drops so low. It's the high level of sugar in the bloodstream and then the rapid plunge (when you finally produce enough insulin) that causes your sharp food cravings. The cravings cause you to eat more carbs, and so the vicious cycle goes around and around.

All of the above is a good explanation for why obesity makes you overeat, and why eating carbs, rather than satisfying your hunger, makes you hungry for more. But we still haven't answered this question: What do obesity and type 2 diabetes or prediabetes have to do with heart trouble?

Effects on the Heart

It starts with that central obesity. Your expanding midsection is not due to an increase in the *number* of fat cells in there. No, when you're overweight, the number of cells remains more or less constant, but each cell increases in size. In other words, the fat cells themselves grow fat. When these cells expand, the insulin has trouble attaching to them properly and unlocking them. That's why, if you weigh too much, the sugar and fat levels in your bloodstream rise higher than they should. The insulin key takes longer to open the lock.

That in turn brings about several other blood conditions, all of which are further signs of type 2 diabetes (and even prediabetes), signs that can be seen only by a doctor. They're a familiar list if you've been paying attention to health news over the past decade: High blood pressure, high triglycerides, low good cholesterol, high ratio of total cholestrol to good, and the relatively unknown but critical matter of too-small bad cholesterol particles.

When insulin isn't working properly, it takes longer than it should to store the fat you just ate. Because of that delay, your liver is being flooded with fatty acids. In response to that, the organ emits harmful particles that deposit fat and cholesterol in the blood vessels of your heart—future blockages, in other words.

So this, then, is the link between obesity and heart disease. The danger isn't the carbs or the sugars themselves. It's how they affect your body's ability to process fats. Eating too many jelly doughnuts may not cause a heart attack. But it can and does create the conditions that will lead to one. Obesity itself doesn't damage your cardiovascular system. It's just the number-one sign of an unhealthy blood profile, which will someday almost certainly curtail your good health, and maybe your life.

Today, alarmingly, we're seeing type 2 diabetes in young adults and even in adolescents. It's not that we're genetically less healthy than previous generations. But our habits are much worse. Gym memberships and home treadmills are staples of middle-class life, but the truth is that we perform less physical activity than our parents and grandparents did. Maybe their jobs required more exertion, or they enjoyed fewer labor-saving devices. Perhaps they just walked a lot more than we do.

This lack of exercise extends even to the youngest among us. I am distressed by the levels of physical playtime children now get. The trends of building schools without schoolyards—which also means no recess—and of cutting phys ed in favor of more classroom instruction are disasters in the making. Time spent in front of the TV, videogames, and computers has not helped.

Probably more harmful than decreasing exercise, however, is how food has changed. As we delegate more and more of our food preparation to fast food restaurants and food manufacturers, its quality has deteriorated—not just in its taste but in its fiber and nutrient content. In a sense, food manufacturers have begun the digestion process for us. Until quite recently we did not appreciate that processed foods were bad and have contributed to our epidemic of obesity. We endured hunger once; now the plenty we enjoy as a nation translates directly into the load on our dinner plates. The fact that more than half of all restaurant meals come in the form of fast-food has only worsened things. Once, the carbs we ate were less processed than they are today. More of our bread was baked at home or in local bakeries, not factories, and was made with whole grains, not flour that had been overly processed and stripped of all fiber. Back then, convenience and speedy preparation weren't the highest ideals food aspired to. We were in less of a rush, and home cooking meant starting with raw ingredients. Rice had more of its fiber intact, and had to be cooked slowly. Potatoes weren't sliced and frozen or powdered and bought in a box. Children's after-school snacks weren't limited to what could be microwaved. More of what we ate had shelf lives measured in days, not months and sometimes years!

We didn't require large infusions of sugar in every meal, starting with our breakfast cereal and continuing at every feeding through the late-night snack of pretzels made from pure, processed white flour. We didn't spend quite so much of our time amid food courts and chocolate chip cookie stands and convenience store coolers and Slurpees and Big Gulps and all the rest.

Even the impulse toward healthy eating brought us closer to this unhealthy state. Next time you visit a supermarket, examine the nutritional information on all the "low-fat" products: Invariably, you'll find that processed carbs have been added to replace the fats. Or notice how many breads there are labeled "vitamin-enriched" or "fortified," which means so much of the natural fiber (which contains the vitamins) has been stripped away that some nutrients had to be added back in!

I realize that I'm describing more than any one patient's eating patterns. It's the nutritional state of the union that's to blame for what's happening internally to many millions of us. Usually, the serious damage doesn't show up until you're in your fifties or sixties. But the invisible harm is being done decades earlier, setting the stage for the future catastrophe.

The cure for this, luckily, is the same as the solution to the overweight problem that vexes millions of people who aren't terribly concerned about their future cardiac well-being. It's what I've tried to codify in a sensible, practical, easy-to-remember-and-follow eating plan that the rest of this book is devoted to explaining. But as far as I'm concerned, this is the true goal of any great diet. Looking good on the outside is important, I know. But having beautiful, physically fit blood vessels and healthy blood chemistry as a result makes it that much more important.

MY SOUTH BEACH DIET

JUDY H.: I WENT FROM A SIZE 32 TO A SIZE 18. I'm 55. I'm divorced. About a year or so ago, I weighed 386 pounds.

It runs in my family. On my mother's side, all the parents and their oldest child—but only the oldest child, which includes me—are heavy. I was fairly thin most of my younger years. But after I had my son and daughter, I gained weight, and I would yo-yo up and down. I've been on many diets over the years, and I've always been able to lose weight. Once I lost 100 pounds on a very severe diet. But eventually, I gained it back.

I was never a breakfast person. Wasn't a coffee drinker. I don't smoke, I don't drink. I would eat nothing all morning, not even a snack. And for lunch I would just eat whatever everybody else in my office was having. I didn't put a lot of thought into it. It could be Chinese food, it could be hamburgers. Whatever the girls were ordering. We had a lot of full lunches brought in—pasta was a big thing for me at lunch.

After that I didn't eat again until dinner. No snacks in the afternoon. And then dinnertime was usually meat, vegetable, salad, and a starch. Pasta. Or potatoes. I was never a rice person. But I really liked my other carbs—pizza and sandwiches, too. I would rather eat a sandwich than sit down and have steak and potatoes. Pastry also—I love pastries. Not a candy eater, but I liked my breads and desserts. I wasn't a big soda drinker. I was never really that thirsty—that was another problem.

Everybody said, go to Weight Watchers. Try Jenny Craig. I've tried everything. One day I was talking to one of the girls in our office and I said to her, "Hey, you look great." And she says, "Oh, I'm on this diet I just heard about, Dr. Agatston's diet." So she gave me a copy. And I just took it and ran with it. And I've lost 135 pounds in the year or so since.

But at first when I looked at this diet and I saw that it restricted carbs, I said, "I'll never be able to do it." But then I said, "Well, you *gotta* do it." So I decided: There will be no more bread in the house. No more milk in the house. I must have had 20 boxes of pasta in the kitchen. Threw it all out. I told my daughter, "Look, if you need a sandwich, go buy a roll and make one. I just can't have it lying around here." I got rid of everything, and I never brought it back into the house.

And, still, to this day, I miss my bread—I really do. I would kill to sit down and eat Italian bread with some butter. But I won't do it. Because I know I can't control myself with that stuff. In the past few weeks I found myself close to slipping a little—like wanting just a taste of this or that. Things I wouldn't even think of tasting before. I asked somebody I know at work, "Do you notice me doing anything different?" And he said, "Yes, I do—when we have lunch in the office, before you wouldn't touch one morsel of something that you weren't supposed to have. Now you'll take a spoon or two." So maybe I've slipped a little. But that's good to know. I'm going to have to watch it with carbs for the rest of my life.

The first day wasn't bad. I felt, like, I *have* to do it. This is my last chance. And I started and just stayed on it. I could see the difference the first week. Within 6 weeks I lost 50 pounds. After that, I began to incorporate more fruits and vegetables into my diet, and some mayonnaise in my tuna, things like that. But I stayed away from having even a little bit of cereal or oatmeal. No starches. Now and then, as a treat, I might have allowed myself a little piece of a roll or something. But I stop myself. If I go out, I only go to restaurants where I know I can eat the food. I'm not going to kill myself and sit in an Italian restaurant. I know better. I'll go to a Chinese restaurant if I know they don't use MSG. You can pick out your own fresh meat and vegetables and things and they'll stir-fry them for you. So I go there maybe twice a week. I'm a big seafood person. I'll eat mussels, crab legs, shrimp. They have green beans cooked with oil and garlic. I'll eat a whole plate of them. Iced tea with Sweet'N Low or diet soda. I go home full. That's my treat, twice a week.

And I don't go to any fast-food places at all anymore, because there's really nothing I can have. My only big treat, once a month—I go to McDonald's and get a low-fat fruit yogurt. It has carbs in it, but I have it anyway. See, they don't tell you about the carbs. So it says "low-fat" but there might be sugar in it. The fruit might have been frozen in sugar. They make you believe you're having something healthy, but you're not. You have to read every single ingredient before you buy anything. Like when I go to the supermarket, I buy the sugar-free Popsicles. When I want something sweet, I'll eat them. And if I have a bad night where I really crave something, I might eat three or four of them. But it gets me over that hump. I make sugar-free Jell-O. I buy diet soda. I have one cup of coffee a day, in the morning.

Now I even try to eat breakfast. I'll have Egg Beaters and maybe two slices of bacon. Or I'll take lunchmeat and just roll it up with some low-fat cheese and a sliced tomato. I'm still not a big breakfast person. But I find that it gets the fire burning.

No baked goods. At work, if they bring in tuna on French bread, I might eat a little of the bread with the tuna. But the times I do that are very few and far between. I can't allow myself. Even now, I'm in a little bit of a stall. I've been yo-yo dieting with the same 10 pounds for the last 3 months. I was back home in Pennsylvania for 3 weeks, and I went to a wedding, a birthday party, and Thanksgiving—and I didn't gain anything. At my nephew's wedding I had the salmon, I ate the salad, and that was it. I didn't have any wedding cake.

On Thanksgiving my brother-in-law made me eggplant and I had salad. I didn't have the turkey and stuffing and potatoes and all that. My family's very supportive when I go home. And it felt good when I went back because I hadn't seen them for a while—at one point I lost 60 pounds between visits, and the next time I saw them I had lost 30 more. By the time of my latest visit back home I had dropped about 125 pounds. I was going to meet an old friend from high school for dinner, and he walked right past me. Then he turned around and said, "Judy? You look no different than 25, 30 years ago." I gave him the biggest kiss. I'm still heavy, don't get me wrong, but on this diet I went from a size 32 to a size 18. This is the only diet that has ever really worked for me. ∎

HOW TO EAT
IN A RESTAURANT

Because this diet is designed to be practical and user-friendly, it's easy to stick to the rules even if you dine out often.

This is not usually the case for weight-loss plans, which is why it was so important to us that the South Beach Diet work no matter who does the cooking. The dining-out dilemma was especially painful for people on low-fat regimens. You either had to give the waitstaff the third degree—What are the chicken breasts sautéed in? What exactly is in the vinaigrette?—or you had to bring your own food and hope no one objected. Even if they didn't, there was something sad about seeing healthy adults hovering over their Tupperware containers while their tablemates enjoyed fine dinners.

The overall trend in restaurant food over the past few decades has been toward healthy and fresh. Olive oil is now an American staple. Every day it seems we read more about the benefits of certain fish. Menus include lots of grilled items and few that are fried. As a result, it's not hard to eat out when you're on the South Beach Diet.

Of course, you still have to watch what you're doing, but eating out is a good time to indulge in the things you love most, if only because doing so makes it a little easier to be moderate the rest of the time. There are a few strategies, many of which we've learned from patients, that can help you eat wisely even when you're on the town.

Here's a simple one: Eat something 15 minutes before you arrive at the restaurant. Just a little snack—a protein of some kind. A piece of low-fat cheese is good because you can carry it in your handbag or briefcase. It will begin the process of filling you up so that when it's time to order, you won't do so while feeling ravenous.

I recommend this also because it will help you get beyond the most treacherous part of any restaurant meal: the bread basket. Typically, you arrive, you're hungry, and there it is—fresh, perhaps warm and fragrant, and loaded with bad carbs. It won't really do much to satisfy your hunger, but it will jolt your bloodstream with glucose and set you up for reactive hypoglycemia and cravings for the rest of the evening.

Many people on the diet take the preemptive measure of telling the waiter to skip the bread basket altogether, which is a great idea as long as your fellow diners don't mind. If they do, you can always ask them to take their bread, *then* banish the basket.

Here's another good idea for the moment you arrive: Order soup, preferably a clear broth or consommé. The point of this, besides being filling, is that it extends your eating time. That's a good idea because there's a lag between when your belly begins to fill and when your brain notices it—maybe 20 minutes, the experts say. This fact explains why it's so easy to reach the point where you feel uncomfortably stuffed. Today, when speed is valued in both the preparation and the consumption of food, this is a danger. We eat so fast that we zoom right by the point of satiety and keep feeding ourselves until all of a sudden, we feel like we'll explode.

Starting a meal with broth begins the process of satisfying your hunger and initiates the signals to your brain that you are on the road to fullness. Anything that takes the edge off your hunger now is good, because it will keep you from eating more than you really need in a little while, when the food arrives.

If you peeked inside the bread basket and found a piece of the good, whole grain variety, you may decide to indulge yourself. If you do, dip it in olive oil, which will slow down the absorption of starches and contribute to your feeling of fullness. Believe it or not, bread with oil or even a little butter is better for your diet than bread alone, despite the fact that you're adding calories.

Here's another tip: Go to restaurants serving Mediterranean-style food. I don't just mean Italian—in fact, Italian restaurants can be dangerous because of how pasta and bread tend to dominate the meal. I'm thinking of Greek and Middle Eastern food. These are cuisines that employ lots of olive oil, which is always a plus. You can have hummus (paste made from chickpeas) on pita bread, which is a *big* improvement over white bread and butter, and it's more flavorful, too. You'll find good, whole grains such as tabbouleh and couscous, which take the place of potatoes or rice. And usually, these cuisines rely on spices and condiments rather than sweeteners to make the dishes taste good.

And if you *do* go Italian, try to structure the meal the way they do in Italy—in courses, with a modest serving of *al dente* pasta topped with a healthy tomato sauce, followed by a main course of meat or fish and fresh vegetables, including either leafy green ones like escarole or spinach or crucifers like broccoli, plus a salad dressed in olive oil. In Italy, you don't sit down in front of a huge dish of pasta with a bottomless bread basket and call it dinner. That's why Italians can eat pasta twice a day and not suffer the obesity rates we see in the United States. In many restaurants here you can request a half-order of pasta as your appetizer. If you try this you'll see that it satisfies. It's important to eat enough good fats (the entrée and the olive oil) and good carbs (the vegetables and the salad) to counter the starches in the pasta.

We all tend to assume that restaurants serving Asian food are healthy. The various Asian national diets tend to be heavy on fish and vegetables, light on heavy meats or sweets. But that's not always the case in Asian restaurants in America. One major difference is portion size—we are accustomed to a lot more food on our plates. And because everybody hates waste, we tend to finish what's there. Another significant difference is in the rice. Asians have always used the whole grain, including the fiber, and your digestive system has to work to get at the starch. In this country, and increasingly in many Asian cities, a more processed variety of white rice is used. That change substantially increases the glycemic load of a meal.

Something else you may not realize: MSG, the flavoring agent, is made from beets, which are a healthy vegetable but have a very high glycemic index. They're loaded with sugar, in other words, though it is disguised fairly well in your average Chinese take-out dinner.

Stay away from rice or potatoes in *any* restaurant. Order a double serving of the vegetables instead. And never order anything that's fried. Roasted, broiled, braised, baked, steamed, even sautéed—all right. If there's a sauce, ask for it on the side. That doesn't mean you won't have any, but I guarantee that you'll be satisfied using half of what they would have ladled on.

As for drinks, start with water as soon as you're seated, but feel free to have a glass or two of red wine (which is actually good for your health and not terribly fattening). Avoid appertifs, liquers, or, worst of all, beer. On Phase 3, if you're going to imbibe at a party or other festive occasion, have a drink made with a distilled liquor such as gin or vodka, and don't mix it with a sugary mixer.

For dessert, don't be too hard on yourself. If you eat out four times a week you need to say no most of the time; but if it feels like a special event, make the most of it. If fresh fruit would do the trick, have that. If fruit with ice cream is what you need, that's fine, too. You can ask for them in separate dishes and make your own dessert, using 3 teaspoons of ice cream topped by the fresh fruit. If only the most decadent chocolate cake will suffice, go ahead and order it—along with enough forks for everyone at the table. Have three bites only and eat them as slowly as possible. Then send the rest away with the first passing busboy. Try this experiment at home: Have three bites of any dessert, then stop and put the rest aside for a few minutes. You'll see that it was just as satisfying as eating the whole thing. And you'll still respect yourself in the morning.

Of course, all this presupposes that you're eating in a normal, sit-down restaurant. But the fact is that most American dining out these days is done in fast-food places. It's hard to think of any strategy that might actually help that situation. Everything seems to conspire to deliver the worst meal possible, at least from our perspective.

Start by eliminating all the main attractions. No burgers (too many saturated fats in the meat and the cooking oil, too many carbs in the bun). No fish, either, since the breading and the cooking method make it even more fattening than the burger. No fries (the worst part of the meal from the glycemic index point of view, both the potatoes and the ketchup). No soda, which is pure sugar rush. Look at how fast-food restaurants emphasize their worst fare—even the offer to "supersize" is simply a way to sell you excessive amounts of the cheapest part of the meal, the soda and fries. The emphasis in fast food is on big, sweet, fat, and *fast*—everything that has made obesity such a problem in America today.

If you can visit a fast-food restaurant and limit yourself to salad (with oil and vinegar instead of any other dressing) and plain grilled chicken breast (in the places that serve it), accompanied by water or coffee, you can do all right. Chicken nuggets or fried chicken are bad news. Like the fish, they're a lot of deep-fried bread over a little meat, all of which has been cooked in a trans fatty substance. Otherwise, you can't really eat at these places and follow any sort of healthful diet. That's no surprise, is it?

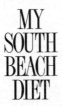

JUDITH W.: I WENT DOWN THREE DRESS SIZES, AND MY CHOLESTEROL IS DOWN, TOO. I've had high blood pressure and angina for many years, and heart trouble runs in my family. I had a triple bypass in 1990, and I was the baby in the cardiac ward. My mother had already had one, and my sister had one, too. A few years ago I needed a new cardiologist and I went to Dr. Agatston. The first thing he told me was that I had to lose weight, and since I weighed 172 at that time I knew he was right. He didn't tell me anything I didn't know. But he gave me the inspiration and he suggested this diet.

I cut out all of the carbs that I was supposed to cut out, and the sugar, too. They told me not to buy no-fat, because that just meant the foods were higher in sugars. But I did buy 2% milk and low-fat cheeses. Before I went on the diet, I never ate breakfast. But I would snack in the evening. I never snacked on sweets; it was always fruit or pretzels. I always ate baked potatoes, but never with butter, because I thought potatoes were all right. I'd have french fries whenever I wanted. Of course, I had a roll with my hamburger. I was trying to eat sensibly, but I wasn't really killing myself at it. And slowly but surely, I gained a lot of weight. I was in a panic when I started the diet, because I had never looked that big in my life. Never.

Once I got through the strict phase, I began adding back some carbs. But not many. I don't trust carbs. I'll eat whole wheat pasta, but just a small amount. Brown rice, too. That's about it. Cheerios. No potatoes at all—only sweet potatoes. I bake them. I won't eat a whole potato, though—half. Sugar-free jams or jellies, if necessary, but I don't have a sweet tooth, so I'm lucky. When I added the carbs back, I still kept losing weight. I will now, occasionally, have a sandwich made with stone-ground whole wheat bread—thin-sliced, if I can get it.

I lost 30 pounds over the course of maybe 6 months, and 3 years later I've kept it all off. I went down three dress sizes, and my cholesterol is down, too. My husband said it's the most expensive diet I ever went on, because I had to throw out all my clothes and start over. I'm an attorney, so I have a very expensive business wardrobe. And we go to a lot of nighttime functions, too. I love it. I finally have a great excuse for a whole new wardrobe now. ▪

BACK TO CARDIOLOGY

As I've noted, I came to study diet and weight loss only via my specialty of preventive cardiology. I fully agree with a quote from the famous Framingham Heart Study group: "A heart attack or stroke should indicate a failure of medical therapy rather than the beginning of medical intervention." I am convinced that preventing most heart attacks and strokes is not a pipe dream but something that is feasible today. Even people who come to me with family histories of premature heart disease can, in most cases, overcome the genetic predisposition. The important thing is to begin prevention early. The earlier it is started, the easier it is to prevent future catastrophe. In too many cases, the first manifestation of heart attack or stroke is also the last.

Diet is, of course, a crucial component of our prevention strategy. For many patients, particularly those with diabetes or prediabetes, it is our primary focus. Exercise is important, and there are wonderful drugs and supplements that figure in to a total health plan. But proper diet is absolutely the most essential element.

If you neglect that, you may someday have to take your chances with the so-called miracles of modern cardiology—angioplasty, coronary artery bypass, transplant, perhaps even the totally artificial heart. Such measures may restore sufficient cardiac function to keep you alive. But you should realize that all these procedures are, implicitly, admissions of failure. These are the extreme, invasive, last-ditch efforts required once the patient and his or her doctors have proven unable to keep the cardiovascular system working as nature intended. In some cases, there's a disease or dysfunction that caused the ailment. Today, the majority of heart attacks and strokes can be *prevented*.

Exercise

As with diet, the goal here should be to find an exercise plan that will seem less like an intervention and more like part of your existing lifestyle— something you can incorporate easily into your routine. You can seek the greatest cardiac workout ever, one that will put you in marathoner shape. But if it requires you to remake your life, it will probably be a flop. You'll never maintain it over the long haul, and the discouragement alone will leave you worse off than before you started.

Besides, you don't really *need* a Marine Corps–level exercise program to have a healthy heart. What you need is a daily dose of activity that will achieve the desired effect as efficiently as possible. Anything beyond that is optional. Too many people approach this as an all-or-nothing proposition. They start out with a high-intensity program, keep it up for a short spell, tire of it, and go back to doing nothing at all. Better to find a 30-minute workout that you'll do daily. You won't burn a lot of calories each session, but the cumulative effect will be beneficial in every way. At the very least you'll offset the pound or two per year that most middle-age people put on without even noticing. Clearly, people who exercise often and with gusto are better off than those who don't. It's not just a matter of cardiac health, either: Moving your body and pushing its limits puts you in a healthy frame of mind, I believe, in addition to the many other benefits.

The first thing you need is some kind of aerobic workout. You don't have to spend an hour on the treadmill, stair machine, elliptical trainer, or running track, however. Here's what I recommend: A brisk 20-minute walk every day. Don't run unless you really want to. Live by this easy-to-remember rule: Breaking a sweat means that you have achieved your goal. You get the majority of benefit from exercise during the first 20 minutes or so. If you want to stop at that point, it's all right. You've achieved your purpose. But you have to do it for 20 minutes, vigorously and religiously, every day. If you like swimming and it's possible to do it year round, be my guest. Again, you don't need to train like an Olympic hopeful. Twenty minutes.

In addition to that, I recommend some stretching, mainly because it ensures that you won't injure yourself doing whatever other exercise you choose. As we age, we lose flexibility. This can be prevented with a good stretching routine.

Finally, weight training has many benefits. It will improve your muscle-to-fat ratio, which will, in turn, raise your metabolism, causing your body to burn fuel faster even when you're asleep. You don't have to become a bodybuilder, but increasing lean body mass—meaning anything other than fat—is important. For women especially, weight training is good for building bone density, which will forestall osteoporosis. Fractured hips and other injuries will be much less likely.

In addition, exercise lowers your blood pressure and increases your good cholesterol. Exercise regularly and eat properly, and you're doing just about all you can to ensure a healthy cardiac future. You're already doing far more for yourself than medical science can do for you.

Before a sustained workout (longer than 90 minutes), it may help to eat some low-glycemic carb, such as low-fat yogurt, oatmeal, or pumpernickel bread. Eat it at least 2 hours before exercising so you'll have a good supply of carbohydrates to give you an energy boost. After exercise, you need to replenish glycogen fuel stores. You may allow yourself white bread or potatoes at this time.

Medications and Supplements

Earlier in the book, I described my journey as a cardiologist firmly committed to the "prevention first" approach, especially as it pertains to diet. But nutrition and exercise alone can't always ensure cardiac health. In the late 1980s a new class of amazing cholesterol-lowering drugs known as the statins—medications such as Mevacor, Pravachol, Lescol, Zocor, and Lipitor—became available. With these, we were able to cut cholesterol quite easily and dramatically—20 to 30 percent initially, and now, up to 50 percent. By taking these drugs, we thought, patients could have their cake and eat it, too—literally. They could diet or not and still enjoy low cholesterol. Of course, statins did nothing for the waistline. Still, the prevailing wisdom was to forget about diet and take the drugs. Statins were (and still are) expensive. However, studies showed that the incidence of heart attacks could be diminished by approximately 30 percent with this class of medications.

I won't burden you with the scientific explanation behind statins. These compounds work by blocking the production of cholesterol in the liver. There has been some controversy associated with them, mainly over the possibility that they cause liver problems. This has been overstated in the popular press. One statin drug, Baycol, was withdrawn from the market because of an unacceptable incidence of toxic reactions. There are only rare problems with the statin drugs now on the market, despite the occasional scare that arises in the papers or on TV news shows. The benefits of statins far outweigh the potential hazards. Among physicians, there has never been any serious doubt about the wisdom of taking them. Consider this: Most cardiologists I know over the age of 40 are taking a statin drug, even doctors with no sign or history of heart trouble. The medication isn't cheap—annual cost is somewhere around $3,000—but the results are worth it.

Supplements, too, have become a big part of cardiac care in recent years.

Most people know to take an aspirin every day to thin the blood slightly and help prevent heart attack and strokes in those at risk. It's worth emphasizing here what a blessing aspirin really is when it comes to cardiac prevention—it's so common and inexpensive that some people forget it's an important part of any heart-healthy regimen.

For years we've been hearing how the classic antioxidant vitamins (A, C, and E) would help prevent heart attack, stroke, and cancer. Recently, though, multiple studies have failed to support these hopes with science. The good news is that current antioxidant vitamins don't do any harm (except to your wallet). The bad news is that they also appear to do no good. There's some evidence that the natural form of vitamin E, called *d*-alpha tocopherol, is effective in preventing heart attacks and strokes. But further study is needed. My advice is to boost your body's supply of antioxidants by exercising and eating fruits and vegetables, which are rich in nutrients. I hedge my bet by suggesting a single daily multivitamin.

In contrast to the antioxidants, the news about taking fish oil supplements, in capsule form is very exciting. Just as we advise people to eat plenty of fish high in beneficial omega-3 oils, such as salmon and tuna, we suggest these capsules. They lower triglycerides and make the blood cells less sticky. They've also been found to prevent sudden death due to cardiac arrhythmia—the sudden, potentially fatal stoppage of the normal heartbeat. Omega-3 supplements also help prevent diabetes and prediabetes. They may also play a role in treating depression and arthritis. (For more on the marvels of fish oil, read Dr. Andrew L. Stoll's excellent book, *The Omega-3 Connection*.)

I, personally, take aspirin, fish oil capsules, and a statin drug.

Recently, a study turned up another potentially important addition to the list of supplements. Some men undergo a kind of menopause equivalent associated with the normal drop in their testosterone levels that begins in their twenties. We've always known that this hormone fuels the sex drive. Now we find that it may also have something to do with cardiac function. Studies indicate that men who have heart attacks often are found to have lower-than-normal testosterone levels. Diabetic men, too, tend to have low testosterone. Replacement of this hormone, when deficient, increases muscle and bone mass and decreases central obesity. It now seems as though the drop in testosterone may be another reason men gain weight as they age.

We never knew any of this before because we measured testosterone only in men with sexual dysfunction. Now we see the impact this hormone has on the entire obesity–cardiac health connection. I test for it in all my male patients and prescribe a testosterone gel (which is rubbed on the skin) for those whose levels are low.

Advanced Blood Testing

Lowering total cholesterol is an important goal in preventive care, but it's not nearly enough. In fact, most people who suffer heart attacks have average cholesterol levels. The fact is that one person can have a low cholesterol number and be at grave risk for a heart attack, while someone else with a higher figure will be fine. The familiar total cholesterol figure *alone* doesn't tell the entire story.

By now, most people realize there are two basic types of cholesterol—the so-called good kind (high-density lipoproteins, or HDLs) and the bad (low-density, or LDLs). The ratio of good-to-bad is an important factor, one that is commonly measured today by diagnostic blood work.

But there are also other factors that must be considered; and for this reason, advanced lipid testing has now become an important addition to cardiac care.

The most sophisticated blood labs are now capable of measuring five different subgroups of HDL and seven of LDL. One thing they evaluate is the *size* of the cholesterol particles. In essence, large particles are good and small ones are bad. Large HDLs have proven to be more efficient at their job of clearing away bad fats than are small HDLs. Even more important, though, is the difference between large and small LDL particles. The small ones squeeze more easily under the lining of blood vessels, where they form the plaque that narrows arteries. Larger LDL particles can't slide beneath the linings as easily; and as a result, their potential for harm is less.

Advanced blood lipid testing has been pioneered by the Lawrence Berkeley National Laboratory of the University of California at Berkeley and its commercial arm, the Berkeley HeartLab. H. Robert Superko, M.D., medical director of the lab, has done an outstanding job of educating doctors in the use of advanced blood testing for treating patients. When the cholesterol subclasses are screened along with other advanced tests, including Lp(a), homocysteine, and others, we can explain over 90 percent of the heart disease we see. We can also test for high sensitivity to C-reactive protein—CRP—a marker for inflammation of the blood vessel lining. Harvard's Paul

Ridker, M.D., did the groundbreaking research proving that inflammation of the arteries can play a big role in arteriosclerosis and heart attacks. Measuring this inflammation can predict who is a candidate for a heart attack, even in patients with normal or low cholesterol. It's interesting to note that people with prediabetes or diabetes often have normal cholesterols but high CRPs.

EBT Scanning

There's a final medical measure that must be taken to promote heart health, one with which I am extremely familiar: electron beam tomography (EBT) as a noninvasive tool for examining the heart. More than the electrocardiograph (EKG) or exercise testing, this technology has the power to tell us the exact condition of the blood vessels that supply the beating heart. This test supplies critical information that no other diagnostic tests provide.

In June of 1988, I worked with my colleagues Warren Janowitz, M.D., David King, and Manuel Viamonte, M.D., to come up with a method of identifying cardiac plaque simply, accurately, and painlessly, without having to invade the body. We used a then-revolutionary type of CT scan called electron beam tomography, or EBT.

This fast, painless (no needles or dye, no undressing) CT scanner was developed by a brilliant physicist, Douglas Boyd, Ph.D. The procedure takes pictures in a fraction of a second, freezing the image of the beating heart. With a conventional CT scanner, the beating heart shows up as a blur. With General Electric's EBT, high resolution of the coronary arteries can be obtained. This allows us to see and measure calcium deposits, which are accurate indicators of the total amount of arteriosclerosis in the vessel walls. Using these images, we can identify who needs to be treated in advance of a heart attack or stroke. By treating the patient with diet, exercise, and medication, we can retest and monitor the effectiveness of the treatment.

Proper diet and exercise are still the most important things you can do to take care of your heart. Combine those with advanced lipid testing, aggressive lipid therapy, and the EBT, and the vast majority of heart attacks and strokes can be prevented.

MY SOUTH BEACH DIET

NANCY A.: I DIDN'T GAIN ANYTHING DURING PREGNANCY. I was working at Mt. Sinai Hospital, in the child care center, where some of the children's parents work in the cardiovascular department. They invited us to be part of some research they were doing, and in exchange we'd get free diet consultations for 3 months. We had to pick a diet at random, and I ended up with the modified carbohydrate diet, which later became known as the South Beach Diet.

When I started I weighed 169 pounds. For the previous 5 years, I had tried everything to lose weight. I tried fen-phen three separate times. That's how I gained so much weight—I gained everything back double every time I stopped. I tried Slim-Fast, too. After a while I was getting really hungry from just drinking shakes, and so I went back to my regular eating habits. On my own, I decided to do salads only. That didn't work, either—I didn't have enough willpower. I would get even hungrier after eating a salad.

I'm Spanish, so we were raised on Spanish foods, which tend to have a lot of fat. I had to cut down on that stuff, fried foods especially. But every time I went a month or two eating healthy foods, I would crave my traditional dishes. Pork in the oven with rice, fried plantains, fried chicken. I couldn't stop myself from wanting it. I'm also a sweets person, so cheesecake here and there, a cookie here and there. I work in a child care center, so we have tons of snacks for the children. After a big dinner, I would eat a bowl of ice cream, or cereal, or cake.

The first 2 weeks on the South Beach Diet were the toughest—just low-fat meats and vegetables and water. Around the second week, I was going crazy. It was psychologically stressful. But I did it. Going to visit the nutritionist was helpful. Within those first weeks I think I cheated once, on cheesecake. A couple times I was tempted to have rice, but I had stopped buying it, so there was none in the house. It kind of killed me, not having it around.

After the 2 strict weeks were up, it got a lot easier. I was able to have more variety. I went to the store and went crazy buying everything that was on the list. I was able to have fruit. And vegetables—I even started eating ones I'd never tried before. I was so eager to have more variety. Broccoli. Asparagus. Anything I saw.

After the 3-month period, I had gotten down from around 170 to 140 pounds. Actually, on the day I made the final visit to the nutritionist, I found out that I was pregnant. And I had been trying for 5 years. In fact, I had given up trying. And here I was, pregnant at last. I don't actually know what triggered that, but I think it's because I had been so over-weight and not eating right. Something must have changed. And I had a perfect pregnancy.

I kept the weight off for 2 years. I didn't gain anything during the pregnancy. And only recently did I start to slide backward. I've been neglecting myself a little, and some of the weight is back on. When you have a 3-year-old and you're working at a day care center, you're sur-rounded by sweets. But I just got another copy of the diet from the nu-tritionist, and I'm going back on it again. ▪

WHY DO PEOPLE OCCASIONALLY FAIL ON THIS DIET?

I t's a good question, because some *do* fail. We're always looking at the reasons, trying to find ways to improve the program. Most people who go on it report that taking the plunge is surprisingly easy. That's partly because the South Beach Diet doesn't require you to give up everything you love. We strongly encourage you to eat until you're no longer hungry, and to snack when you feel the need, even during the stringent first 2 weeks.

But we recognize that it's also easy at the start because it's human nature to be gung-ho at the beginning of *any* new health regimen. You're feeling motivated, and so you're optimistic and full of resolve and determination to get your life and your looks back on track. Before you know it, you're watching the pounds begin to melt away. You see the numbers on your scale descend, and you dig out garments that were once uncomfortably snug—or maybe even impossibly tight—and suddenly they begin to seem possible again. Sticking with the program is easy with so much positive reinforcement.

Then what happens?

To a degree, failure comes because of the program's success. People lose anywhere from 8 to 13 pounds during the first 2 weeks. At that point you switch from the strictest phase to Phase 2, when you begin reintroducing some of the carbs you cut completely in Phase 1. The purpose of adding them back, as I've said, is manifold: Some carbs are good for you, and we want you to be on a healthy diet that's as close to "normal" eating as possible. That means you're going to eat fruit, and bread or pasta once in a while, and even a dessert here and there.

You continue losing weight in Phase 2, but not at the same speed as you did in Phase 1. Depending on how much you want to lose, it may take up to a year or even longer.

For some dieters, that's a disappointment. And they remember that Phase 1 wasn't *so* restrictive. They couldn't eat certain things they love, but they never went hungry or felt discomfort. So they decide to stay on Phase 1 indefinitely, until they reach their goal.

Now, I know plenty of dieters who have made that decision and succeeded. But I know plenty more who have failed.

Here's why they fail: Phase 1 isn't meant to be a long-term eating plan. You're limited to a fairly small palette of foods—grilled or broiled lean meats and fish, vegetables, low-fat cheeses and salads, all either steamed or prepared using good fats such as olive oil and canola oil. For snacks, nuts and part-skim mozzarella sticks, and that's about it.

From a culinary point of view, it's a perfectly acceptable diet—for 2 or 3 weeks. After that, it gets a little dull. That is where the trouble starts.

That's when dieters begin to improvise, only they do so improperly. They mix in their bad old habits—just once in a while, mind you. They follow Phase 1 but they add in a handful of Oreo cookies every night. Even that's not exactly it. They add in one cookie after dinner, realize it tasted pretty good and probably did no harm, and then increase it to three every night. Three cookies a night with no noticeable harm makes it easy to allow a small bag of corn chips at 4 o'clock one afternoon. If you're doing all right with three cookies and corn chips, it doesn't seem so unwise to indulge a craving for pizza and beer on the weekend.

Before long, you're cheating more than dieting.

When you realize how badly you've strayed, you may do what lots of other people have tried: You'll revert at once to the strict Phase 1 plan. But when you do, it seems even more monotonous than it did the first time.

At that point, you may just surrender. Some people do. If you're lucky, you won't end up weighing more than you did before you started the diet, though backsliding has a way of sending you to a point even beyond where you began.

It's a diet truism that you can't lose in a day what took you years to put on. We all accept that, and yet it's hard not to try the quick fix. Sometimes the end result is weight gain, not loss.

It's important for people to like the food they eat. Eating is meant to bring pleasure, even when you're trying to lose weight. That's a sensible way to think about food, and it's one of the basic principles of the South Beach Diet. Which is why we strongly urge all the people we counsel to switch to Phase 2 after the second week, no matter how tempting it is to remain on Phase 1. This is a long-term diet, and the three-phase approach is an important part of its success. It may take longer to lose the weight this way, but your chances of losing it and keeping it off are better.

Daily Challenges

A second reason for failure has more to do with how everyday life intrudes on our plans. You've reached your target weight. Now you're in Phase 3, the diet's maintenance stage, meaning you still have to eat a certain way to *keep* the weight off. If you stick with the program, this is how you'll eat for the rest of your life.

What kind of intrusions am I talking about? People who travel a good deal, especially on business, are at a high risk for diet failure. Travel is disruption, especially of your normal eating routines. That's dangerous. It's especially so nowadays when in-flight food service has become a thing of the past. Once, you could plan ahead and order the special vegetarian or kosher meal and you'd get something fresh and healthy and made to order. You could easily bypass the meat with gravy, mashed potatoes, peas and carrots, applesauce, and fruit cobbler for dessert.

Today, more than likely all you've been served is some trail mix or honey-roasted peanuts with soda. Except for the nuts, it's all carbs and sugars.

By the time you've landed and made it to your hotel, it's way past your mealtime. With the change in time zones, it may even be past your bedtime. But you're wired from the trip, and famished. The first thing you do is pick up the room service menu and overorder—maybe a Caesar salad with roast chicken breast would be enough to satisfy your hunger, but you hear yourself requesting the turkey club sandwich with french fries and a milk shake. You regret the decision as soon as you hang up the phone, but when the food arrives you somehow manage to force it all down, along with a beer from the minibar to make you drowsy enough to sleep.

The next day you eat properly, but as you near your normal dinnertime you're stuck in a working session at the home office. It's not until 7:30—when you're starving once again—that somebody thinks to order in a few pizzas and soft drinks. And so you end another day loaded with bad carbs.

Long workdays, whether at home or on the road, are a main culprit in diet failure. It's the disruption of normal mealtimes that leads you to overeat when the food finally arrives. Or you're one of those modern-day road warriors, a businessperson or sales rep who spends hours in a car grabbing an unhealthy lunch or snack at a fast-food drive-through window and wolfing it down in the parking lot.

Sometimes it's the work-related stress that makes it easy to fall back into comforting old habits. People who eat when they feel psychological or emotional pressure tend to fall off the diet wagon. Think of the items we call comfort foods—invariably it's either baked sweets, like cakes and pies and chocolate chip cookies, or dishes such as macaroni and cheese.

I can't tell you how many people went off the diet in the fall and winter of 2001. The terrorist attacks jarred us out of our sense of safety, or they made weight seem like an awfully trivial concern in the larger scheme of things. That's the kind of anxiety and insecurity that seeks comfort in a sweet mouthful or a brimming dinner plate. It's hard to advise people how to cope with that kind of stress while sticking to a diet.

Elsewhere in this book I've included testimonials from people who have gone on the South Beach Diet, gotten down to their desired weight, and remained there. Here I'm going to quote someone who went on the diet, lost weight, and then backslid—so much so that today he weighs pretty much what he did when he started. His story is a good example of how, sometimes, just a momentary break in the diet can spell disaster. In its way, this should be as instructive as the others. To protect the guilty, though, I won't name this dieter.

I had had an early heart attack—I'm in my fifties—and was in cardiac rehab when I finally decided it was time to lose weight. I was up around 235 at the time. I went to the nutritionist, and she set me up on a 4-week version of the South Beach Diet.

In the first 2 weeks I lost about 8 pounds. But it left me feeling a little weak. Then I started adding back some carbs, and I felt better, and the weight kept coming off. Bread was my big weakness back then. I ate it with every meal, and sometimes I ate it between meals. If I went to a restaurant I'd feast on the bread basket, to the point where I wouldn't be hungry when dinner came. I'd have to take it home many times. So I cut the bread out completely.

My other big weakness was sweets. I love cookies, especially oatmeal raisin. I'd eat them all day long—I'd buy them fresh baked and take them into work for everyone, but I'd grab a handful every time I walked by the kitchen.

I had always eaten a lot of potatoes, too, and I had to give them up, but it wasn't too hard. Bread and cookies were the tough ones. Waffles, too, with syrup, for breakfast. Or a Danish. After I went on the diet, I cut out all the baked goods from my breakfast and just stuck with eggs. Lots of water to drink, and decaf.

Instead of cookies between meals, I'd have nuts. Maybe some peanuts in the middle of the afternoon. And no more dessert at night.

Before, I'd have more cookies, or maybe a big bowl of cereal with milk. On the diet I had almonds for my dessert, while I was watching TV. I'd count 15 of them out of the jar like I was told, and I'd eat them slowly, one by one, so they'd last.

On Phase 2, I lost another 25 pounds. And it was getting easier. At restaurants I'd ask them to take the bread away. I'd stick with meat and vegetables and felt just fine.

Then, the way you're supposed to, I started adding some carbs back to my diet. I'd have a slice of bread every couple of days, for instance, or instead of bread I'd have a serving of rice. I kept losing weight, and I stayed with the diet for a whole year.

That's about when we had a big family outing to attend. A huge party. I had been good for so long that I said to myself I was going to eat anything and everything I wanted. I told myself that it would just be for one day, and that tomorrow I'd go back on the program.

But tomorrow never came. I liked eating everything so much I didn't want to stop. In the past, if I added too many carbs and stopped losing weight, I'd just shift back on Phase 1 and take it off. This time I couldn't bring myself to do it. Before I knew it, all the weight I had lost—almost 50 pounds—was back. Now I'm planning to go back to Phase 1 again, but it'll be starting all over. This is a very good diet, and it really works. But you still have to actually *follow* it."

It's true that this particular dieter could easily have indulged his sweet tooth all day long at the family picnic, and the next morning gone back on the diet. That's how plenty of people operate: They'll give in to temptation on special occasions—a wedding, say, or on vacation, or at a fancy dinner—and then make up for it the next day. On this diet you can fall off the wagon, find that you've put on a pound or two, and easily backtrack to Phase 1 until you lose what you've gained.

All this makes perfect sense, of course—even to the people who fall off the wagon so hard that they undo weeks and even months of good work. It's okay to fall off once in a while, as long as you remember to get right back on!

MY SOUTH BEACH DIET

STEVE L.: IF YOU FALL OFF THE WAGON OCCASIONALLY, YOU HOP BACK ON. I had begun seeing Dr. Agatston as my cardiologist when we moved down here. My first appointment with him was in his office—not in an exam room—where he pulled out his laptop and went through a little PowerPoint presentation and said, "If we decide to work together, this is what our cardiac disease prevention protocol is like. And if you have a heart attack, then I've failed."

Bad hearts run in my family, so it was important to me to get this under control. I've always been an athletic guy. I'm a fairly big guy, a little over six two. And when I started this I was probably about 270 pounds—which was my heaviest. I can hide it fairly well, and I can move comfortably with the weight, but it wasn't too healthy. And I'm from Minnesota—it's a meat-and-potatoes and high-carb lifestyle.

My huge weaknesses are bread and pasta. We moved down here from Seattle, where we had a pizza oven in our kitchen. So all my cravings were about carbs. Not sweets. But everything else. If we went to a restaurant, I could easily handle the bread basket by myself. I'd have bread a minimum of three times a day. And while I'm not a dessert guy, there would always be cookies around.

Part of the problem also was a fair amount of ignorance on my part. I grew up under the impression that all fruits were healthy. Then I learned that some are high in sugar and some aren't. I didn't realize, for instance, that watermelon is full of sugar, whereas cantaloupe is not. Eggs, on the other hand, have moved into the positive category. I'm not a big drinker but I used to drink beer. I haven't had a beer for 2-plus years.

My wife and I love to cook—and we love to eat. But we started having brown rice instead of white and sweet potatoes instead of regular ones. Root vegetables, frankly, weren't that difficult for me to give up. We've discovered some really great recipes, and we grill like crazy. A lot of grilled vegetables. And much more fish than we used to eat. Bread only in limited quantities. I'll have half a bagel for breakfast. If I decide to have a sandwich for lunch, it's with either rye or pumpernickel, and it's less bread and more meat than before.

I'd gone on diets my whole life, and usually at the outset I got the heebie-jeebies, and lightheadedness, all that stuff. On this, I felt abso-lutely fine. No side effects. I stopped caffeine for 2 weeks, too, and I'm a coffee hog. My wife had an enormously difficult time the first 2 weeks. But for me it was nothing. And we were strict. I mean, I would go to work with some pistachios and a part-skim cheese stick for the afternoon snack. There are some pretty good low-fat cheeses. The huge, trau-matic thing for me was bread.

In the 6 months I've been on the diet, I've lost about 50 pounds. I put some of that back on due to stress eating lately, but I know I can go back to the strict phase and lose it again. And with Dr. Agatston's blessing, if there's something we feel an urgent craving for, we just go have it. If you fall off the wagon occasionally, you hop back on. So if we go out to dinner, we'll order dessert once in a while—maybe one time out of three. But just one dessert for the two of us, and we'll take a bite or two each and then send it away. Just enough to end the meal on a sweet taste. And I drink red wine only—no other alcohol. Not only have I lost the weight, but all my numbers are improved. My triglycerides, for example, went from 256 to 62 after 6 weeks. And that was all diet. Cho-lesterol numbers continue to move down. ▪

PART TWO

Meal Plans and Recipes

PHASE
ONE
Meal Plan

This, as you know by now, is the strictest phase of the diet. It's meant to last for 2 weeks only—just long enough to resolve the insulin resistance that was brought about by eating too many bad (mostly processed) carbs. Phase 1 does not have to be *low* carb if you eat the *right* carbs. It is designed to allow ample portions of protein, good fats, and and the lowest glycemic index carbs needed for satisfaction and blood sugar control. These include the low-glycemic index vegetables, which also contribute fiber, important nutrients such as heart-healthy folate, and other vitamins and minerals. Many salads and vegetables are unlimited. You will also have your choice of proteins from a variety of sources.

By the time this phase ends, your unhealthy cravings, especially for sweets, baked goods, and starches, will have essentially vanished. You'll notice that each day includes six different occasions to eat. So you should never feel hungry, and if you do, it's possible that you're being too stingy with your portions. The South Beach Diet doesn't require you to measure what you eat in ounces, calories, or anything else. The meals should be of normal size—enough to satisfy your hunger, but no more than that.

Day 1

Breakfast

6 oz vegetable juice cocktail

2 Vegetable Quiche Cups to Go (page 134)

Decaffeinated coffee or decaffeinated tea with nonfat milk and sugar substitute

Midmorning snack

1 part-skim mozzarella cheese stick

Lunch

Sliced grilled chicken breast on romaine

2 Tbsp Balsamic Vinaigrette (page 148) or low-sugar prepared dressing

Sugar-free flavored gelatin dessert

Midafternoon snack

Celery stuffed with 1 wedge Laughing Cow Light Cheese

Dinner

Grilled Salmon with Rosemary (page 162)

Steamed asparagus

Tossed salad (mixed greens, cucumbers, green peppers, cherry tomatoes)

Olive oil and vinegar to taste or 2 Tbsp low-sugar prepared dressing

Dessert

Vanilla Ricotta Crème (page 181)

Day 2

Breakfast

6 oz tomato juice

¼–½ cup liquid egg substitute

2 slices Canadian bacon

Decaffeinated coffee or decaffeinated tea with nonfat milk and sugar substitute

Midmorning snack

1–2 Turkey Roll-Ups (page 179)

2 Tbsp Cilantro Mayonnaise (optional) (page 179)

Lunch

South Beach Chopped Salad with Tuna (page 140)

Sugar-free flavored gelatin dessert

Midafternoon snack

Celery stuffed with 1 wedge Laughing Cow Light Cheese

Dinner

Baked chicken breast

Roasted Eggplant and Peppers (page 169)

Tossed salad (mixed greens, cucumbers, green peppers, cherry tomatoes)

2 Tbsp Balsamic Vinaigrette (page 148) or low-sugar prepared dressing

Dessert

Mocha Ricotta Crème (page 182)

Day 3

Breakfast

6 oz vegetable juice cocktail

Easy Asparagus and Mushroom Omelet (page 132)

Decaffeinated coffee or decaffeinated tea with nonfat milk and sugar substitute

Midmorning snack

1 part-skim mozzarella cheese stick

Lunch

Dilled Shrimp Salad with Herb-Dill Dressing (page 142)

Sugar-free flavored gelatin dessert

Midafternoon snack

1–2 Ham Roll-Ups (page 179)

2 Tbsp Cilantro Mayonnaise (optional) (page 179)

Dinner

Broiled sirloin steak

Steamed broccoli

Broiled Tomatoes (page 173)

Surprise South Beach Mashed "Potatoes" (page 171)

Dessert

Almond Ricotta Crème (page 181)

Day 4

Breakfast

6 oz tomato juice

Eggs Florentine (1 poached egg served on ½ cup spinach sautéed in olive oil)

2 slices Canadian bacon

Decaffeinated coffee or decaffeinated tea with nonfat milk and sugar substitute

Midmorning snack

Celery stuffed with 1 wedge Laughing Cow Light Cheese

Lunch

Chef's salad (at least 1 oz each ham, turkey, and low-fat cheese on mixed greens)

Olive oil and vinegar to taste or 2 Tbsp low-sugar prepared dressing

Midafternoon snack

Up to 10 cherry tomatoes stuffed with ½ cup low-fat cottage cheese

Dinner

Orange Roughy in Scallion and Ginger Sauce (page 163)

Steamed snow peas

Shredded cabbage sautéed in olive oil

Dessert

Mocha Ricotta Crème (page 182)

Day 5

Breakfast

6 oz vegetable juice cocktail

Western Egg White Omelet (page 133)

Decaffeinated coffee or decaffeinated tea with nonfat milk and sugar substitute

Midmorning snack

1–2 Turkey Roll-Ups (page 179)

2 Tbsp Cilantro Mayonnaise (optional) (page 179)

Lunch

Gazpacho (page 149)

Grilled sirloin hamburger steak (no bun)

Tossed salad (mixed greens, cucumbers, green peppers, cherry tomatoes)

Olive oil and vinegar to taste or 2 Tbsp low-sugar prepared dressing

Midafternoon snack

Cucumber rounds with salmon spread

Dinner

Balsamic Chicken (page 151)

Stewed Tomatoes and Onions (page 172)

Steamed spinach

Tossed salad (mixed greens, cucumbers, green peppers, cherry tomatoes)

Olive oil and vinegar to taste or 2 Tbsp low-sugar prepared dressing

Dessert

Almond Ricotta Crème (page 181)

Day 6

Breakfast

6 oz tomato juice

Scrambled eggs with fresh herbs and mushrooms

2 slices Canadian bacon

Decaffeinated coffee or decaffeinated tea with nonfat milk and sugar substitute

Midmorning snack

1 part-skim mozzarella cheese stick

Lunch

Chicken Caesar salad (no croutons)

2 Tbsp prepared Caesar dressing

Midafternoon snack

½ cup low-fat cottage cheese with ½ cup chopped tomatoes and cucumbers

Dinner

Mahi mahi

Oven-Roasted Vegetables (page 168)

Arugula salad

2 Tbsp Balsamic Vinaigrette (page 148) or low-sugar prepared dressing

Dessert

Lemon Zest Ricotta Crème (page 180)

Day 7

Breakfast

6 oz vegetable juice cocktail

Smoked Salmon Frittata (page 131)

Decaffeinated coffee or decaffeinated tea with nonfat milk and sugar substitute

Midmorning snack

Celery stuffed with 1 wedge Laughing Cow Light Cheese

Lunch

Crab Cobb Salad (page 143)

Sugar-free flavored gelatin dessert

Midafternoon snack

2 slices low-fat mozzarella cheese with 2 slices fresh tomato sprinkled with balsamic vinegar, olive oil, and freshly ground black pepper

Dinner

Marinated London Broil (page 158)

Spinach-Stuffed Mushrooms (page 170)

Surprise South Beach Mashed "Potatoes" (page 171)

Tossed salad (mixed greens, cucumbers, green peppers, cherry tomatoes)

Olive oil and vinegar to taste or 2 Tbsp low-sugar prepared dressing

Dessert

Lime Zest Ricotta Crème (page 182)

Day 8

Breakfast

Light Spinach Frittata with Tomato Salsa (page 130)

Decaffeinated coffee or decaffeinated tea with nonfat milk and sugar substitute

Midmorning snack

1 part-skim mozzarella cheese stick

Lunch

Sliced steak (leftover London broil) on mixed greens

2 Tbsp Balsamic Vinaigrette (page 148) or 2 Tbsp low-sugar dressing

Sugar-free flavored gelatin dessert

Midafternoon snack

Hummus (page 178) with raw vegetables

(May use store-bought hummus)

Dinner

Savory Chicken Sauté (page 153)

Surprise South Beach Mashed "Potatoes" (page 171)

Fresh steamed green beans

Boston lettuce and pecan salad

Olive oil and vinegar to taste

Dessert

Vanilla Ricotta Crème (page 181)

Day 9

Breakfast

6 oz vegetable juice cocktail

2 Vegetable Quiche Cups to Go (page 134)

Decaffeinated coffee or decaffeinated tea with nonfat milk and sugar substitute

Midmorning snack

1–2 Turkey Roll-Ups (page 179)

2 Tbsp Cilantro Mayonnaise (optional) (page 179)

Lunch

Greek Salad (page 137)

Sugar-free flavored gelatin dessert

Midafternoon snack

Celery stuffed with 1 wedge Laughing Cow Light Cheese

Dinner

Fish Kabobs (page 166)

Oven-Roasted Vegetables (page 168)

Sliced English cucumber with olive oil

Dessert

Lemon Zest Ricotta Créme (page 180)

Day 10

Breakfast

6 oz tomato juice

Egg white omelet with chopped Canadian bacon and mushrooms

Decaffeinated coffee or decaffeinated tea with nonfat milk and sugar substitute

Midmorning snack

1 wedge Laughing Cow Light Cheese

Lunch

Salad Niçoise (page 147)

Midafternoon snack

½ cup low-fat cottage cheese

Dinner

Cracked Pepper Steak (page 160)

Broiled Tomato with Pesto (page 173)

Steamed broccoli

Mixed field greens

2 Tbsp Balsamic Vinaigrette (page 148) or low-sugar prepared dressing

Dessert

Almond Ricotta Crème (page 181)

Day 11

Breakfast

6 oz tomato juice

Cheesy Frittata (page 129)

Decaffeinated coffee or decaffeinated tea with nonfat milk and sugar substitute

Midmorning snack

1–2 Turkey Roll-Ups (page 179)

2 Tbsp Cilantro Mayonnaise (optional) (page 179)

Lunch

Gazpacho (page 149)

Grilled sirloin hamburger steak (no bun)

Tossed salad (mixed greens, cucumbers, green peppers, cherry tomatoes)

Olive oil and vinegar to taste or 2 Tbsp low-sugar prepared dressing

Midafternoon snack

Fresh mozzarella cheese balls

Dinner

Gingered Chicken Breast (page 152)

Steamed snow peas

Oriental Cabbage Salad (page 177)

Dessert

Almond Ricotta Crème (page 181)

Day 12

Breakfast

6 oz vegetable juice cocktail

Broccoli and Ham Frittata (page 131)

Decaffeinated coffee or decaffeinated tea with nonfat milk and sugar substitute

Midmorning snack

1 wedge Laughing Cow Light Cheese

Lunch

Chicken-Pistachio Salad (page 141)

Midafternoon snack

Fresh mozzarella cheese balls

Dinner

Poached Salmon with Cucumber Dill Sauce (page 161)

Edamame Salad (page 176)

Broiled Tomatoes (page 173)

Steamed asparagus

Dessert

Lemon Zest Ricotta (page 180)

Day 13

Breakfast

Baked eggs in Canadian bacon cups

Decaffeinated coffee or decaffeinated tea with nonfat milk and sugar substitute

Midmorning snack

Celery stuffed with 1 wedge Laughing Cow Light Cheese

Lunch

Poached Salmon Spinach Salad (poached salmon left over from Day 12) (page 161)

Olive oil and vinegar to taste or 2 Tbsp low-sugar prepared dressing

Midafternoon snack

Hummus (page 178) with raw vegetables

(May use store-bought hummus)

Dinner

Grilled Steak with Grilled Tomato Relish (page 159)

Dessert

Mocha Ricotta Crème (page 182)

Day 14

Breakfast

Artichokes Benedict (page 135)

Mock Hollandaise Sauce (page 136)

Decaffeinated coffee or decaffeinated tea with nonfat milk and sugar substitute

Midmorning snack

1–2 Turkey Roll-Ups (page 179)

2 Tbsp Cilantro Mayonnaise (optional) (page 179)

Lunch

Cottage cheese and chopped vegetables in red pepper cup

Midafternoon snack

Hummus (page 178) with raw vegetables

(May use store-bought hummus)

Dinner

Grilled chicken breast with grilled vegetables and fennel or endive

Dessert

Sugar-free flavored gelatin dessert with a tablespoon fat-free frozen whipped topping or whipping cream with sugar substitute to taste

FOODS TO ENJOY

BEEF
Lean cuts, such as:
Sirloin (including ground)
Tenderloin
Top round

POULTRY (SKINLESS)
Cornish hen
Turkey bacon (2 slices per day)
Turkey and chicken breast
Low-fat turkey sausage (one serving per week)

SEAFOOD
All types of fish and shellfish

PORK
Boiled ham
Canadian bacon
Tenderloin

VEAL
Chop
Cutlet, leg
Top round

LUNCHMEAT
Fat-free or low-fat only

CHEESE (FAT-FREE OR LOW-FAT)
American
Cheddar
Cottage cheese, 1–2% or fat-free
Cream cheese substitute, dairy-free
Feta
Mozzarella
Parmesan
Provolone
Ricotta
String

NUTS
Almonds, 15
Cashews, 15
Macadamias, 8
Peanut butter, 2 Tbsp

Peanuts, 20 small
Pecan halves, 15
Pistachios, 30

EGGS
The use of whole eggs is not limited unless otherwise directed by your doctor. Use egg whites and egg substitute as desired.

DAIRY
Milk, fat-free or 1%
Milk, soy, plain low-fat (4 g of fat or less per serving)
Buttermilk, fat-free or 1%
Yogurt, plain fat-free

TOFU
Use soft, low-fat or lite varieties that contain 3 grams of fat or less per 2–3 oz serving

VEGETABLES AND LEGUMES
Artichokes
Asparagus
Beans
Broccoli
Cabbage
Cauliflower
Celery
Collard greens
Cucumbers
Eggplant
Lettuce (all varieties)
Mushrooms (all varieties)
Snow peas
Spinach
Sprouts, alfalfa
Tomatoes
Turnips
Water chestnuts
Zucchini

FATS
Oil, canola and olive

SPICES AND SEASONINGS

All spices that contain no added sugar
Broth
Extracts (almond, vanilla, or others)
Horseradish sauce
I Can't Believe It's Not Butter! Spray
Pepper (black, cayenne, red, white)

SWEET TREATS (LIMIT TO 75 CALORIES PER DAY)

Candies, hard, sugar-free
Chocolate powder, no sugar added
Cocoa powder, baking type
Fudgsicles, no sugar added
Gelatin, sugar-free
Gum, sugar-free
Popsicles, sugar-free
Sugar substitute

FOODS TO AVOID

BEEF

Brisket
Liver
Other fatty cuts
Rib steaks

POULTRY

Chicken, wings and legs
Duck
Goose
Poultry products, processed

PORK

Honey-baked ham

VEAL

Breast

CHEESE

Brie
Edam
Nonreduced fat

VEGETABLES

Beets
Carrots
Corn
Potatoes, white
Potatoes, sweet
Yams

FRUIT

Avoid all fruits and fruit juices in Phase 1, including:
Apples
Apricots
Berries
Cantaloupe
Grapefruit
Peaches
Pears

STARCHES AND CARBS

Avoid all starchy food in Phase 1, including:
Bread, all types
Cereal
Matzo
Oatmeal
Rice, all types
Pasta, all types
Pastry and baked goods, all types

DAIRY

Avoid the following dairy in Phase 1:
Yogurt, cup-style and frozen
Ice cream
Milk, whole or 2%

MISCELLANEOUS

Alcohol of any kind

PHASE
ONE
Recipes

Because this is the strictest phase, the palette of ingredients is relatively small. You'll be eating eggs and egg substitutes for breakfast and lots of vegetables, low-fat cheeses, meat, and fish the rest of the time. There's no bread, potatoes, fruit, or rice during the first 2 weeks, true. But any plan that permits dishes such as Marinated Flank Steak, Crab Cobb Salad, Hummus, and Lemon Zest Ricotta Crème can hardly be termed tough. And any program that requires you to eat six times a day—three meals plus snacks in midmorning and midafternoon, plus a nighttime dessert—is clearly meant to keep discomfort to a minimum.

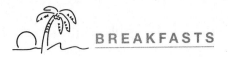 **BREAKFASTS**

Cheesy Frittata

    2 teaspoons Smart Balance spread
    ½ cup sliced onion
    ½ cup sliced red bell pepper
    ½ cup sliced zucchini
    2 small plum tomatoes, diced
    1 tablespoon chopped fresh basil
       Pinch freshly ground black pepper
    ½ cup liquid egg substitute
    ½ cup 1% cottage cheese
    ¼ cup fat-free evaporated milk
    ¾ ounce shredded reduced-fat Monterey Jack cheese

Coat an ovenproof 10" skillet with cooking spray and place over
medium-low heat until hot. Melt the spread in the skillet. Add the onion,
bell pepper, and zucchini and sauté over medium-low heat until the
vegetables are lightly browned, 2–3 minutes. Add the tomatoes, basil, and
black pepper to the skillet and stir to combine. Cook until the flavors are
blended, 2–3 minutes, and remove from the heat.

 Preheat the broiler. In a blender, combine the egg substitute, cottage
cheese, and milk and process until smooth. Pour the egg mixture over the
vegetables. Cover and cook on medium-low heat until the bottom is set
and the top is still slightly wet. Transfer the skillet to the broiler and broil
until the top is set, 2–3 minutes. Sprinkle with the shredded cheese and
broil until the cheese melts.

Serves 2

NUTRITION AT A GLANCE

Per serving: 231 calories, 21 g protein,
16 g carbohydrates, 10 g fat, 3 g saturated fats,
480 mg sodium, 15 mg cholesterol, 2 g fiber

Light Spinach Frittata with Tomato Salsa

Frittata

- 1 tablespoon extra-virgin olive oil
- 1 small onion, sliced
- 2 cloves garlic, minced
- 1 package (10 ounces) frozen spinach, thawed and well-drained
- 2 large eggs
- 3 egg whites
- ⅓ cup fat-free evaporated milk
- ½ cup shredded reduced-fat mozzarella cheese

Salsa

- 4 plum tomatoes, seeded and chopped
- 2 scallions , minced
- 1 clove garlic, minced
- 2 tablespoons minced fresh cilantro
- 1 tablespoon fresh lime juice
- ¼ teaspoon salt
- ⅛ teaspoon freshly ground black pepper

To make the frittata: Preheat the oven to 350°F. Heat the oil in a 10" nonstick skillet over medium heat. Add the onion and garlic and cook, stirring, for 3 minutes or until tender. Stir in the spinach. Reduce the heat to low. In a large bowl, beat the eggs and egg whites with the milk until light yellow and frothy. Pour the egg mixture over the spinach in the skillet. Cook for 5–7 minutes, until the egg mixture is cooked on the bottom and almost set on top. Sprinkle with the cheese. Bake in the oven until the eggs are set and the cheese has melted, 5–10 minutes.

To make the salsa: In a large bowl, stir together the tomatoes, scallions, garlic, cilantro, lime juice, salt, and pepper. Serve fresh, at room temperature, over the frittata.

You can also serve the frittata with commercial jarred salsa.

Serves 2

NUTRITION AT A GLANCE

Per serving: 369 calories, 27 g protein, 28 g carbohydrates, 17 g fat, 6 g saturated fats, 740 mg sodium, 230 mg cholesterol, 8 g fiber

Smoked Salmon Frittata

8 stalks fresh asparagus

1 tablespoon extra-virgin olive oil

½ Bermuda onion

¼ cup dry-packed sun-dried tomatoes

2 ounces smoked salmon

½ cup liquid egg substitute

¼ cup water

3 tablespoons nonfat dry milk

¼ teaspoon chopped fresh marjoram

Pinch freshly ground black pepper

fat-free sour cream (optional)

salmon roe (optional)

chives (optional)

Boil 1" of water in a large skillet. Add the asparagus and cook, uncovered, until tender-crisp. Coat an ovenproof 8" skillet with cooking spray and place over medium-low heat until hot. Add the olive oil and sauté the onion until soft. Add the asparagus and sun-dried tomatoes. Add the smoked salmon and remove from the heat.

Preheat the broiler. Combine the egg substitute, water, dry milk, marjoram, and pepper. Pour over the salmon mixture. Cover and cook over medium-low heat for 7 minutes or until the bottom is set and the top is slightly wet. Place the skillet under the broiler 4"–6" from the heat source until the top of the frittata is puffed and set, 2–3 minutes. Top with fat-free sour cream, salmon roe, marjoram, and chives, if desired. Slice into wedges and serve immediately.

Try substituting 1 cup of broccoli florets for the asparagus and 2 ounces of ham for the salmon.

Serves 2

NUTRITION AT A GLANCE

Per serving: 241 calories, 19 g protein,
18 g carbohydrates, 11 g fat, 2 g saturated fats,
730 mg sodium, 5 mg cholesterol, 4 g fiber

Easy Asparagus and Mushroom Omelet

3 stalks fresh asparagus

2 eggs

2 tablespoons water

¼ cup sliced white mushrooms

¼ cup shredded reduced-fat mozzarella cheese

Boil 1" of water in a large skillet. Add the asparagus and cook, uncovered, just until tender-crisp.

Meanwhile, in a medium bowl, whisk together the eggs and water until the whites and the yolks are completely blended.

Coat a 10" nonstick skillet with cooking spray. Heat the skillet over medium-high heat until just hot enough to sizzle when a drop of water is added. Pour in the egg mixture. It should set immediately.

With an inverted pancake turner, lift the edges as the mixture begins to set to allow the uncooked portion to flow underneath.

When the top is set, fill one half of the omelet with the asparagus, mushrooms, and cheese.

With the pancake turner, fold the omelet in half over the filling. Slide onto a serving plate. Serve immediately.

Serves 1

NUTRITION AT A GLANCE

Per serving: 238 calories, 21 g protein,
5 g carbohydrates, 15 g fat, 6 g saturated fats,
260 mg sodium, 440 mg cholesterol, 1 g fiber

Western Egg White Omelet

1 tablespoon chopped green bell pepper

1 tablespoon chopped scallion

1 tablespoon chopped red bell pepper

½ cup liquid egg substitute

3 tablespoons shredded reduced-fat cheese

Lightly coat a medium skillet with cooking spray. Sauté the peppers and the scallions until they are tender-crisp. Pour the egg substitute over the vegetables. When partially set, spread the cheese over half of the egg substitute and fold the omelet in half over the filling. Continue cooking until cooked through. Serve immediately.

Serves 1

NUTRITION AT A GLANCE

Per serving: 169 calories, 20 g protein, 4 g carbohydrates, 8 g fat, 3 g saturated fats, 320 mg sodium, 15 mg cholesterol, 1 g fiber

Vegetable Quiche Cups To Go

1 package (10 ounces) frozen chopped spinach

¾ cup liquid egg substitute

¾ cup shredded reduced-fat cheese

¼ cup diced green bell peppers

¼ cup diced onions

3 drops hot-pepper sauce (optional)

Microwave the spinach for 2½ minutes on high. Drain the excess liquid.

Line a 12-cup muffin pan with foil baking cups. Spray the cups with cooking spray.

Combine the egg substitute, cheese, peppers, onions, spinach, and hot-pepper sauce (if using) in a bowl. Mix well. Divide evenly among the muffin cups. Bake at 350°F for 20 minutes, until a knife inserted in the center comes out clean.

Quiche cups can be frozen and reheated in the microwave. Any combination of appropriate vegetables and reduced-fat cheeses may be used.

Serves 6

NUTRITION AT A GLANCE

Per serving: 77 calories, 9 g protein,
3 g carbohydrates, 3 g fat, 2 g saturated fats,
160 mg sodium, 10 mg cholesterol, 2 g fiber

Artichokes Benedict

2 medium artichokes

2 slices Canadian bacon

2 eggs

4 tablespoons Mock Hollandaise Sauce (see page 136)

Wash the artichokes. Cut off the stems at the base and remove the small bottom leaves. Stand the artichokes upright in a deep saucepan filled with 2"–3" of salted water. Cover and boil gently, 35–45 minutes. Turn the artichokes upside down to drain.

Spread the leaves open like flower petals. With a spoon, carefully remove the center petals and the fuzzy center from the artichoke bottoms and discard. Keep the artichokes warm.

Brown the Canadian bacon in a skillet and poach the eggs in boiling salted water. Place a bacon slice into each artichoke. Top with a poached egg and 2 tablespoons of Mock Hollandaise Sauce. Serve immediately.

Serves 2

NUTRITION AT A GLANCE

Per serving: 227 calories, 18 g protein,
16 g carbohydrates, 12 g fat, 3 g saturated fats,
540 mg sodium, 225 mg cholesterol, 8 g fiber

Mock Hollandaise Sauce

¼ cup liquid egg substitute

1 tablespoon Smart Balance spread

1 teaspoon fresh lemon juice

½ teaspoon Dijon mustard

Dash ground red pepper

In a 1-cup microwaveable liquid measure, combine the egg substitute and the spread. Microwave on low (20%) for 1 minute, stirring once halfway through cooking, until the spread is softened.

Stir the lemon juice and mustard into the egg substitute mixture. Microwave on low for 3 minutes, stirring every 30 seconds, until thickened. Stir in the pepper.

If the mixture curdles, transfer to a blender and process on low speed for 30 seconds, until smooth.

Serves 2

NUTRITION AT A GLANCE

Per serving: 54 calories, 4 g protein,
2 g carbohydrates, 4 g fat, 0 g saturated fats,
150 mg sodium, 5 mg cholesterol, 0 g fiber

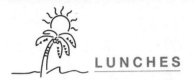

LUNCHES

Greek Salad

8 leaves romaine lettuce, torn into bite-size pieces

1 cucumber, peeled, seeded, and sliced

1 tomato, chopped

½ cup sliced red onion

½ cup crumbled reduced-fat feta cheese

2 tablespoons extra-virgin olive oil

2 tablespoons fresh lemon juice

1 teaspoon dried oregano leaves

½ teaspoon salt

Combine the lettuce, cucumber, tomato, onion, and cheese in a large bowl.

Whisk together the oil, lemon juice, oregano, and salt in a small bowl. Pour over the lettuce mixture and toss until coated.

This makes a nice accompaniment as a side salad for grilled chicken or fish.

Serves 1

NUTRITION AT A GLANCE

Per serving: 501 calories, 22 g protein,
25 g carbohydrates, 38 g fat, 10 g saturated fats,
2,300 mg sodium, 30 mg cholesterol, 6 g fiber.
Greek salad w/out salt: 1,134 mg sodium

From the Menu of ...

1220 AT THE TIDES

1220 Ocean Drive, Miami Beach

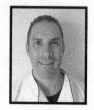

EXECUTIVE CHEF: ROGER RUCH

LOCATED ON OCEAN DRIVE, THE CRITICALLY ACCLAIMED 1220 AT THE TIDES RESTAURANT IS ADJACENT TO THE LOBBY IN THE BEAUTIFULLY RESTORED TIDES HOTEL. CHEF ROGER RUCH CREATES CULINARY MASTERPIECES IN A CASUAL YET LUXURIOUS SETTING. THE TIDES' SOPHISTICATED ELEGANCE MAKES IT A FAVORITE OF THE LOCALS AS WELL AS VISITORS TO SOUTH BEACH.

Cherry Snapper Ceviche

4 cherry snapper (tilapia) fillets, medium dice

Juice of 3 fresh limes

½ teaspoon red chili garlic paste (sambal oelek)

2 ripe Roma tomatoes, medium dice

½ yellow Spanish onion, medium dice

2½ tablespoons fresh cilantro, finely chopped

Kosher salt

Black pepper

Soak the diced fish in ¾ of the lime juice for 3 hours. Drain off the liquid and discard.

Mix the fish with the red chili garlic paste, tomatoes, onion, cilantro, and the remaining lime juice. Season with salt and pepper to taste.

The fish is cooked by the lime's acidity rather than by heat.

Serves 4

NUTRITION AT A GLANCE
Per serving: 225 calories, 36 g protein, 15 g carbohydrates, 2 g fat, 1 g saturated fats, 115 mg sodium, 63 mg cholesterol, 3 g fiber

South Beach Chopped Salad with Tuna

Salad

1 can (6 ounces) water-packed tuna

⅓ cup chopped cucumber

⅓ cup chopped tomato

⅓ cup chopped avocado

⅓ cup chopped celery

⅓ cup chopped radishes

1 cup chopped romaine lettuce

Dressing

4 teaspoons extra-virgin olive oil

2 tablespoons fresh lime juice

2 cloves garlic, finely chopped

½ teaspoon black pepper

To make the salad: Layer the tuna, cucumber, tomato, avocado, celery, radishes, and lettuce in a decorative glass bowl.

To make the dressing: Mix the olive oil, lime juice, garlic, and pepper. Drizzle over the salad.

Serves 1

NUTRITION AT A GLANCE

Per serving: 506 calories, 48 g protein, 18 g carbohydrates, 28 g fat, 4 g saturated fats, 640 mg sodium, 50 mg cholesterol, 6 g fiber

Chicken-Pistachio Salad

Salad

½ cup shelled pistachio nuts, finely ground

½ + ¼ teaspoon salt

½ teaspoon + 1 pinch freshly ground black pepper

4 boneless, skinless chicken breast halves

2 tablespoons extra-virgin olive oil

½ cup diced sweet white onion

1 head romaine lettuce

Dressing

1 teaspoon grated sweet white onion

1 large ripe avocado, pitted and peeled

3 tablespoons extra-virgin olive oil

3 tablespoons fresh lime juice

1 tablespoon water

To make the salad: Preheat the oven to 375°F. Mix the nuts in a pie plate with ½ teaspoon salt and ½ teaspoon pepper. Press the chicken into the nuts. Heat 1 tablespoon of the oil in a skillet and cook the coated breasts, 2 minutes per side. Place the breasts in a baking dish and bake for 15 minutes or until a thermometer inserted in the thickest portion registers 160°F and the juices run clear.

Heat the remaining tablespoon of oil in a nonstick skillet over high heat. Add the diced onion, ¼ teaspoon salt, and a pinch of pepper. Cook until the onion is browned.

Line 4 serving plates with lettuce. Slice the chicken breasts and arrange 1 breast on top of the lettuce on each plate. Serve with the dressing.

To make the dressing: Puree the onion, avocado, oil, lime juice, and water in a blender.

Serves 4

NUTRITION AT A GLANCE

Per serving: 481 calories, 33 g protein, 13 g carbohydrates, 34 g fat, 5 g saturated fats, 520 mg sodium, 70 mg cholesterol, 5 g fiber

Dilled Shrimp Salad with Herb-Dill Dressing

Shrimp

- 1 cup dry white wine
- 1 teaspoon mustard seeds
- ¼ teaspoon red-pepper flakes
- 2 bay leaves
- 1 lemon, sliced
- 1½ pounds large shrimp, peeled and deveined
- 4 ripe tomatoes, cut into wedges
- 6 fresh mushrooms, sliced

  Fresh dill sprigs (optional)

Herb-Dill Dressing

- 3 tablespoons extra-virgin olive oil
- 3 tablespoons red wine vinegar
- 2 tablespoons water
- 2 tablespoons chopped fresh basil
- 2 tablespoons chopped fresh dill
- 1 teaspoon finely chopped garlic
- 1 teaspoon Dijon mustard
- ½ medium onion, sliced
- 1 large head romaine lettuce

To make the shrimp: Combine the wine, mustard seeds, pepper flakes, bay leaves, and lemon in a large saucepan. Add water to fill the pan two-thirds full. Bring to a boil over high heat. Add the shrimp, and cook for 3–4 minutes or until the shrimp have turned pink and are no longer translucent in the center. Drain and cool. Discard the bay leaves.

To make the herb-dill dressing: In a screw-top jar, mix the olive oil, red wine vinegar, water, basil, dill, garlic, mustard, and onion. Shake well.

Place the shrimp in a large bowl and add the dressing. Toss well, cover, and refrigerate until well-chilled.

Serve the shrimp mixture on romaine lettuce leaves and surround with the tomato wedges and mushroom slices. Garnish with dill sprigs, if using.

Serves 4

NUTRITION AT A GLANCE

Per serving: 382 calories, 38 g protein,
16 g carbohydrates, 14 g fat, 2 g saturated fats,
310 mg sodium, 260 mg cholesterol, 4 g fiber

Crab Cobb Salad

6   cups romaine lettuce, torn into bite-size pieces

1   can crabmeat (6 ounces), drained

1   cup ripe tomatoes or cherry tomatoes, halved

¼   cup crumbled blue cheese

2   tablespoons cholesterol-free bacon bits

¼   cup prepared low-sugar dressing or olive oil vinaigrette

Chill 2 plates.

Arrange the lettuce on a large serving platter. Arrange the crabmeat, tomatoes, blue cheese, and bacon bits in rows over the lettuce.

Right before serving, drizzle some dressing evenly over the salad and toss well. Transfer to the 2 chilled plates.

Serves 2

NUTRITION AT A GLANCE

Per serving: 267 calories, 27 g protein,
12 g carbohydrates, 13 g fat, 4 g saturated fats,
1,012 mg sodium, 95 mg cholesterol, 4 g fiber

From the Menu of . . .

CHINA GRILL

404 Washington Avenue, Miami Beach

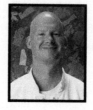

CHEF: **CHRISTIAN PLOTCZYK**

A WILDLY SUCCESSFUL SPINOFF OF THE ACCLAIMED CHINA GRILL IN NEW YORK, THIS IS A SOUTH BEACH HOT SPOT. WHILE ASIAN FLAVORS AND TECHNIQUES ARE AN INFLUENCE, CHINA GRILL PROVIDES AN EXCITING DINING EXPERIENCE THAT GATHERS INGREDIENTS FROM AROUND THE GLOBE. GO WITH A GROUP; DISHES ARE MEANT TO BE SHARED.

Spicy Tuna

2   ounces white pepper

2   ounces black pepper

2   ounces fennel seeds

2   ounces coriander seeds

2   ounces ground cumin

2   tuna fillets (8 ounces each)

4   egg yolks

¼   bunch cilantro

¼ bunch chives

¼ bunch parsley

4 seeded jalapeños (wear plastic gloves when handling)

8 ounces mirin (rice vinegar)

12 ounces olive oil

3 roasted red peppers

1 cucumber, finely sliced

Preheat the oven to 325°F. Roast the white pepper, black pepper, fennel, and coriander for 15 minutes. Mix with the cumin and process all of the spices in a blender until finely ground.

Coat the tuna well with the roasted spices, and pan sear until medium-rare. Set aside.

In a blender, make a jalapeño vinaigrette by mixing 2 of the egg yolks with the cilantro, chives, parsley, and jalapeños and 4 ounces of the mirin. Slowly add 6 ounces of oil to emulsify.

In a blender, make a roasted pepper vinaigrette by mixing the remaining 2 egg yolks with the remaining 4 ounces of rice vinegar and the roasted red peppers. Emulsify with the remaining oil.

Pour the jalapeño vinaigrette and the roasted pepper vinaigrette on each half of a large platter. Slice the tuna and place on top of the vinaigrettes. Garnish with the cucumber slices.

Since eggs are unpasturized, you may want to substitute a liquid pasturized egg product (like Egg Beaters). One-quarter cup of liquid egg substitute is the equivalent of 1 whole egg.

Serves 4

NUTRITION AT A GLANCE
Per serving: 626 calories, 37 g protein, 57 g carbohydrates, 26 g fat,
4 g saturated fats, 137 mg sodium, 266 mg cholesterol, 21 g fiber

Mixed Greens with Crabmeat Salad

2 cups torn curly endive

2 cups loosely packed watercress leaves

2 cups torn fresh spinach

2 cups torn red leaf cabbage

½ cup sliced water chestnuts

½ cup julienne-sliced red bell pepper

12 ounces crabmeat, fresh or canned

    Joe's Mustard Sauce (page 174)

Combine the endive, watercress, spinach, cabbage, water chestnuts, and pepper in a large bowl. Toss well. Add the crabmeat.

Divide between 4 serving plates. Drizzle Joe's Mustard Sauce on top.

Serves 4

NUTRITION AT A GLANCE

Per serving: 123 calories, 20 g protein,
9 g carbohydrates, 1 g fat, 0 g saturated fats,
338 mg sodium, 76 mg cholesterol, 4 g fiber

Salad Niçoise

½ pound tiny green beans

½ pound tiny ripe tomatoes, cut into wedges

1 green bell pepper, seeded and cut into strips

1 English cucumber, cut into thick strips

2 ounces canned anchovies, drained

½ cup pitted black olives

7 ounces water-packed canned tuna, drained and flaked

½ cup sliced water chestnuts

4 hard-cooked eggs, quartered

5 tablespoons extra-virgin olive oil

1 tablespoon white wine vinegar

1 clove garlic, minced

Pinch salt

Pinch freshly ground black pepper

2 tablespoons finely chopped flat-leaf parsley

Blanch the beans briefly until tender-crisp and refresh in cold running water. Pat dry.

Mix the tomatoes, pepper, and cucumber in a large salad bowl (or place in separate piles around the inside of the bowl). Arrange the anchovies, olives, tuna, water chestnuts, and eggs over the top.

Make a dressing by vigorously mixing the oil, vinegar, and garlic with the salt and pepper. Pour the dressing over the salad and sprinkle with the parsley.

Serves 4

NUTRITION AT A GLANCE

> **Per serving:** 405 calories, 26 g protein,
> 14 g carbohydrates, 27 g fat, 5 g saturated fats,
> 1,010 mg sodium, 240 mg cholesterol, 4 g fiber

Balsamic Vinaigrette

⅓ cup extra-virgin olive oil

⅓ cup balsamic vinegar

2 teaspoons chopped fresh thyme

¼ teaspoon salt

⅛ teaspoon white pepper

1 tablespoon chopped fresh basil

Combine the olive oil, vinegar, thyme, salt, pepper, and basil in a screw-top jar. Cover and shake.

Makes ⅔ cup

NUTRITION AT A GLANCE

Per serving: 90 calories, 0 g protein,
2 g carbohydrates, 9 g fat, 1 g saturated fats,
75 mg sodium, 0 mg cholesterol, 0 g fiber

Gazpacho

2½ cups tomato or vegetable juice

1 cup peeled, seeded, finely chopped fresh tomatoes

½ cup finely chopped celery

½ cup finely chopped cucumber

½ cup finely chopped green bell pepper

½ cup finely chopped green onion

3 tablespoons white wine vinegar

2 tablespoons extra-virgin olive oil

1 large clove garlic, minced

2 teaspoons finely chopped fresh flat-leaf parsley

½ teaspoon salt

½ teaspoon Worcestershire sauce

½ teaspoon freshly ground black pepper

Combine the juice, tomatoes, celery, cucumber, bell pepper, onion, vinegar, oil, garlic, parsley, salt, Worcestershire sauce, and black pepper in a large glass or stainless steel bowl. Cover and refrigerate overnight.

Serve cold.

Serves 5

NUTRITION AT A GLANCE

Per serving: 117 calories, 2 g protein,
13 g carbohydrates, 6 g fat, 1 g saturated fats,
690 mg sodium, 0 mg cholesterol, 4 g fiber

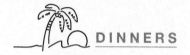 **DINNERS**

Chicken en Papillote

4   boneless, skinless chicken breast halves (about 1 pound)

Pinch salt

Pinch freshly ground black pepper

2   scallions, chopped

1   medium carrot, sliced diagonally

1   small zucchini, cut lengthwise in half, then crosswise into ½" pieces

1   teaspoon dried tarragon

½   teaspoon grated orange zest

Heat oven to 400°F (425°F if foil is used). Cut four 2-foot lengths of parchment paper or foil. Fold each in half to make a 1-foot square. Sprinkle the chicken breasts with salt and pepper. Place a breast slightly below the middle of each square of paper.

In a small bowl, combine the scallions, carrot, zucchini, tarragon, and orange zest. Spoon ¼ of the vegetable mixture over each chicken breast.

Fold the parchment or foil over the chicken and crimp the edges together tightly. Bake for 20 minutes on a baking sheet.

To serve, cut an X in the top of each packet with scissors and tear to open.

Serves 4

NUTRITION AT A GLANCE

Per serving: 144 calories, 27 g protein,
4 g carbohydrates, 2 g fat, 0 g saturated fats,
86 mg sodium, 65 mg cholesterol, 1 g fiber

Balsamic Chicken

6 boneless, skinless chicken breast halves

1½ teaspoons fresh rosemary leaves, minced, or ½ teaspoon dried

2 cloves garlic, minced

½ teaspoon freshly ground black pepper

½ teaspoon salt

2 tablespoons extra-virgin olive oil

4–6 tablespoons white wine (optional)

¼ cup balsamic vinegar

Rinse the chicken and pat dry. Combine the rosemary, garlic, pepper, and salt in a small bowl and mix well. Place the chicken in a large bowl. Drizzle with the oil, and rub with the spice mixture. Cover and refrigerate overnight.

Preheat the oven to 450°F. Spray a heavy roasting pan or iron skillet with cooking spray. Place the chicken in the pan and bake for 10 minutes. Turn the chicken over. If the drippings begin to stick to the pan, stir in 3–4 tablespoons water or white wine (if using).

Bake about 10 minutes or until a thermometer inserted in the thickest portion registers 160°F and the juices run clear. If the pan is dry, stir in another 1–2 tablespoons of water or white wine to loosen the drippings. Drizzle the vinegar over the chicken in the pan.

Transfer the chicken to plates. Stir the liquid in the pan and drizzle over the chicken.

Serves 6

NUTRITION AT A GLANCE

Per serving: 183 calories, 26 g protein,
4 g carbohydrates, 6 g fat, 1 g saturated fats,
270 mg sodium, 65 mg cholesterol, 0 g fiber

Gingered Chicken Breast

1   tablespoon fresh lemon juice

1½ teaspoons grated fresh ginger

½   teaspoon freshly ground black pepper

2   cloves garlic

4   boneless, skinless chicken breast halves

Combine the lemon juice, ginger, pepper, and garlic in a small bowl.

Place the chicken breasts in a deep bowl. Pour the ginger mixture over the breasts, turning once to coat both sides. Cover, and refrigerate for 30 minutes to 2 hours.

Spray a large nonstick skillet with cooking spray. Heat the skillet on medium-high until hot. Add the chicken. Cook, turning once, until tender, about 8 minutes.

Serves 4

NUTRITION AT A GLANCE

Per serving: 129 calories, 26 g protein,
1 g carbohydrates, 1 g fat, 0 g saturated fats,
75 mg sodium, 65 mg cholesterol, 0 g fiber

Savory Chicken Sauté

2 tablespoons extra-virgin olive oil

4 boneless, skinless chicken breast halves

1 large onion, sliced

2 cloves garlic, minced

1 tablespoon fresh rosemary leaves, chopped

½ cup fat-free chicken broth

Pinch salt

Pinch freshly ground black pepper

Heat the oil in a large skillet over medium heat. Sauté the chicken breasts in the oil for 4 minutes, then turn them over and add the onion. Cover and cook for 3 minutes longer, stirring occasionally. Add the garlic, rosemary, and broth. Cover and cook until the onion is tender-crisp, about 5 minutes longer, stirring occasionally. Season with salt and pepper.

Serves 4

NUTRITION AT A GLANCE

Per serving: 217 calories, 28 g protein, 6 g carbohydrates, 8 g fat, 1 g saturated fats, 95 mg sodium, 65 mg cholesterol, 1 g fiber

From the Menu of . . .

TUSCAN STEAK

431 Washington Avenue, Miami Beach

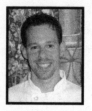

CHEF: MICHAEL WAGNER

TUSCANY, WHERE THE FOOD IS SIMPLE, USUALLY GRILLED, AND
CONSISTENTLY DELICIOUS, HAS FOUND ITS WAY TO SOUTH
BEACH AT TUSCAN STEAK. BEST DESCRIBED AS "A
SOPHISTICATED FAMILY-STYLE FLORENTINE GRILL FEATURING
TUSCAN CUISINE WITH FLORIDA ACCENTS," THERE'S NOTHING
QUITE LIKE TUSCAN STEAK.

Florentine-Style T-Bone

3½ pounds prime T-bone steak

⅓ cup minced fresh garlic

1 cup chopped parsley

1 cup chopped basil

Salt

Freshly ground black pepper

1 cup extra-virgin olive oil

Pinch salt

Pinch freshly ground black pepper

Season the steak with the garlic, parsley, and basil. Add salt and pepper to taste. Drizzle the steak with the olive oil and marinate for 24 hours.

When ready to cook, heat the grill and cook the steak for 1 hour over medium heat, turning every 10 minutes. While grilling, preheat the oven to 400°F. When the meat is ready, remove it from the grill and let it stand for 20 minutes. Roast the meat in the oven for 10-to-30 minutes, depending on how you like it. One hour on the grill and 10 minutes in the oven yields a medium-rare meat. A meat thermometer should register 145°F for medium-rare.

Slice the steak and drizzle it with olive oil.

Serves 4

NUTRITION AT A GLANCE
Per serving: 885 calories, 59 g protein, 5 g carbohydrates, 68 g fat, 13 g saturated fats, 170 mg sodium, 105 mg cholesterol, 1 g fiber

Marinated Flank Steak

1   small red onion, quartered

⅓   cup balsamic vinegar

¼   cup capers, drained

2   tablespoons chopped fresh oregano

3   cloves garlic, minced

1½   pounds flank steak

¼   teaspoon salt

¼   teaspoon coarsely ground black pepper

Sliver one-quarter of the onion and set aside. Chop the rest of the onion. Mix it in a bowl with the vinegar, capers, oregano, and garlic. Combine ¼ cup of this mixture with the slivered onions and set aside.

Sprinkle both sides of the steak with the salt and pepper; prick well with a fork. In a large zip-top food-storage bag, combine the steak with the remaining onion mixture. Marinate for 1 hour or overnight.

Heat the grill or the broiler, positioning the oven broiler rack so that the meat on the rack in the pan is 4" from the heat source. Remove the meat from the marinade, and place on the grill over direct heat or on an oven rack set in the broiler pan. Discard the marinade. Grill or broil for 4–5 minutes per side for medium-rare. Let stand for 5 minutes before slicing.

Place the meat on a platter and pour the reserved onion mixture over the steak.

Serves 6

NUTRITION AT A GLANCE

Per serving: 176 calories, 19 g protein,
3 g carbohydrates, 9 g fat, 4 g saturated fats,
230 mg sodium, 50 mg cholesterol, 1 g fiber

Broiled Flank Steak

1 flank steak (1½ pounds)

½ cup tomato juice

¼ cup Worcestershire sauce

1 small onion, finely chopped (¼ cup)

1 tablespoon fresh lemon juice

1 clove garlic, minced

½ teaspoon freshly ground black pepper

⅛ teaspoon salt

Place the steak in a 13" x 9" glass baking dish. Combine the tomato juice, Worcestershire sauce, onion, lemon juice, garlic, pepper, and salt. Pour the mixture over the steak. Cover and refrigerate for 2 hours, turning once.

Place the steak on the broiler rack and brush with the marinade. Broil 3" from the heat for 5 minutes. Turn, brush with the marinade, and broil for 3 minutes or until a thermometer inserted in the center registers 145°F (for medium-rare).

To serve, cut diagonally across the grain into thin slices.

Serves 4

NUTRITION AT A GLANCE

Per serving: 265 calories, 29 g protein, 6 g carbohydrates, 13 g fat, 6 g saturated fats, 440 mg sodium, 70 mg cholesterol, 0 g fiber

Marinated London Broil

2   tablespoons extra-virgin olive oil

½   cup dry red wine

3   cloves garlic, minced

3   tablespoons minced fresh parsley

1   tablespoon chopped fresh oregano

1   bay leaf

½   teaspoon freshly ground black pepper

1½   pounds sirloin, top round, or eye round London broil

In a small mixing bowl, whisk together the oil, wine, garlic, parsley, oregano, bay leaf, and pepper. Place the steak in a deep bowl and pour on the marinade. Turn once to coat both sides, cover, and refrigerate for at least 4 hours, preferably overnight.

When ready to serve, preheat the broiler or prepare a charcoal grill. Discard the marinade and bay leaf. Broil the meat for about 5 minutes on each side or until a thermometer inserted in the center registers 145°F (for medium-rare).

Cut the meat into thin, diagonal slices across the grain. Serve warm or cold.

Serves 8

NUTRITION AT A GLANCE

Per serving: 171 calories, 17 g protein,
1 g carbohydrates, 10 g fat, 3 g saturated fats,
50 mg sodium, 40 mg cholesterol, 0 g fiber

Grilled Steak with Grilled Tomato Relish

2 sirloin steaks (6 ounces each)

2 medium pear-shaped tomatoes, halved lengthwise

2 tablespoons extra-virgin olive oil

1 medium onion, chopped

1 clove garlic, minced or pressed

¼ cup chopped fresh basil or 2 tablespoons dry basil

Pinch salt

Pinch freshly ground black pepper

Basil sprigs (optional)

Place the steak on a lightly greased grill 4"–6" above a solid bed of medium-hot coals. Cook, turning as needed, until evenly browned on the outside and a thermometer inserted in the center registers 145°F (for medium-rare). Cut to test for doneness (about 15 minutes).

Meanwhile, place the tomatoes on the grill, cut sides up, and brush them lightly with 1 tablespoon of the oil. When the tomatoes are browned on the bottom (about 3 minutes), turn them over and continue to cook until soft when pressed (about 3 more minutes).

While the tomatoes are grilling, combine the remaining 1 tablespoon of oil, the onion, and garlic in a medium frying pan with a heatproof handle. Set the pan over the coals (or set on the stove over medium-high heat). Cook, stirring often, until the onion is soft and golden (about 10 minutes). Stir in the basil.

When the tomatoes are soft, stir them into the onion mixture, then set the pan aside on a cooler area of the grill (or cover and keep warm on the stove).

When the steak is done, place it on a board with a well (or on a platter). Spoon the tomato relish alongside the steak. Season with the salt and pepper and garnish with basil sprigs, if using.

To serve, cut the meat into thin slices. Combine the accumulated meat juices with the tomato relish, if desired.

Serves 2

NUTRITION AT A GLANCE

Per serving: 366 calories, 31 g protein,
11 g carbohydrates, 22 g fat, 5 g saturated fats,
70 mg sodium, 85 mg cholesterol, 3 g fiber

Cracked Pepper Steak

1 tablespoon cracked black pepper

½ teaspoon dried rosemary

2 beef tenderloins, 1" thick (4–6 ounces each)

1 tablespoon Smart Beat spread

1 tablespoon extra-virgin olive oil

¼ cup brandy or dry red wine

Combine the pepper and the rosemary in a large bowl. Coat both sides of the steak with the mixture.

Heat the Smart Beat and oil in a skillet until hot. Add the steaks and cook over medium to medium-high heat for 5–7 minutes or until a thermometer inserted in the center registers 160°F (for medium).

Remove the steaks from the skillet and cover to keep them warm.

Add the brandy to the skillet and bring to a boil over high heat, scraping particles from the bottom of the skillet. Boil for about 1 minute or until the liquid is reduced by half. Spoon the sauce over the steaks.

Serves 2

NUTRITION AT A GLANCE

Per serving: 322 calories, 24 g protein,
3 g carbohydrates, 21 g fat, 6 g saturated fats,
55 mg sodium, 70 mg cholesterol, 1 g fiber

Poached Salmon with Cucumber-Dill Sauce

Salmon

2 cups Chablis or other dry white wine

2 cups water

½ teaspoon chicken-flavored bouillon granules

6 peppercorns

4 sprigs fresh dillweed

2 bay leaves

1 rib celery, chopped

1 small lemon, sliced

6 salmon fillets, ½" thick (4 ounces each)

Cucumber-Dill Sauce

⅓ cup peeled, seeded, finely chopped cucumber.

⅓ cup fat-free sour cream

⅓ cup fat-free plain yogurt

2 teaspoons chopped fresh dill-weed

1 teaspoon Dijon mustard

Fresh dillweed sprigs (optional)

To make the salmon: Combine the wine, water, bouillon, peppercorns, dillweed, bay leaves, celery, and lemon in a skillet. Bring to a boil; cover, reduce heat, and simmer for 10 minutes. Add the salmon to the mixture in the skillet and cook for 10 minutes or until the fish flakes easily.

Transfer the salmon to a platter, using a slotted spoon. Cover, and chill thoroughly. Discard the liquid mixture remaining in the skillet.

To make the cucumber-dill sauce: In a medium bowl, mix together the cucumber, sour cream, yogurt, dillweed, and mustard.

To serve, place the fillets on individual serving plates. Spoon the sauce evenly over the fillets. Garnish with fresh dillweed sprigs, if using.

Serves 6

NUTRITION AT A GLANCE

Per serving: 260 calories, 24 g protein, 5 g carbohydrates, 13 g fat, 3 g saturated fats, 150 mg sodium, 70 mg cholesterol, 0 g fiber

Grilled Salmon with Rosemary

- 1 pound salmon
- 2 teaspoons extra-virgin olive oil
- 2 teaspoons fresh lemon juice
- ¼ teaspoon salt
  Pinch freshly ground black pepper
- 2 cloves garlic, minced
- 2 teaspoons fresh rosemary leaves, chopped, or 1 teaspoon dried, crushed
  Capers (optional)
  Fresh rosemary sprigs (optional)

Cut the fish into 4 equal-size portions. Combine the olive oil, lemon juice, salt, pepper, garlic, and rosemary in a bowl. Brush the mixture onto the fish.

To grill, arrange the fish on a grill rack or use a grill basket sprayed with olive oil cooking spray. Grill over medium-hot coals until the fish flakes easily (allow 4–6 minutes per ½" of thickness). If the fish is more than 1" thick, gently turn it halfway through grilling.

To broil, spray the rack of a broiler pan with olive oil cooking spray and arrange the fish on it. Broil 4" from the heat for 4–6 minutes per ½" of thickness. If the fish is more than 1" thick, gently turn it halfway through broiling.

To serve, top the fish with capers, if using, and garnish with rosemary sprigs, if desired.

Serves 4

NUTRITION AT A GLANCE

Per serving: 231 calories, 23 g protein,
1 g carbohydrates, 15 g fat, 3 g saturated fats,
213 mg sodium, 67 mg cholesterol, 0 g fiber

Orange Roughy in Scallion and Ginger Sauce

⅓ cup dry sherry or vermouth

3 tablespoons reduced-sodium soy sauce

2 teaspoons sesame oil

¼ cup finely chopped green onion

1 teaspoon freshly grated ginger

1 teaspoon finely chopped garlic

2 orange roughy fillets (1 pound)

Preheat the oven to 400°F. Mix the sherry or vermouth, soy sauce, sesame oil, onion, ginger, and garlic in a small bowl.

Place the fish fillets in an ovenproof casserole dish. Drizzle the mixture over the fish and bake for 12 minutes or until the fish flakes easily.

Cod, sole, or flounder may be substituted for the orange roughy.

Serves 2

NUTRITION AT A GLANCE

Per serving: 242 calories, 35 g protein, 3 g carbohydrates, 6 g fat, 1 g saturated fats, 1,154 mg sodium, 45 mg cholesterol, 1 g fiber

From the Menu of ...

JOE'S STONE CRAB

11 Washington Avenue, Miami Beach

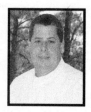

EXECUTIVE CHEF: **ANDRE BIENVENUE**

In 1913, Joe Weiss opened a small lunch counter on Miami Beach. For 90 years, no visit to Miami Beach has been complete without a stop at Joe's. Open during stone crab season (October 15–May 15), Joe's is a must for visiting celebrities. Still family owned and operated, Joe's is a Miami landmark.

Armand Salad

1 or 2	small cloves garlic
¼	teaspoon salt
½	teaspoon pepper
1	teaspoon mayonnaise
¼–½	cup fresh lemon juice
1	teaspoon red wine vinegar (optional)
¼	cup + 2 tablespoons olive oil

1   head romaine lettuce, outer leaves removed, washed, dried, torn into bite-size pieces, and chilled

1   small head iceberg lettuce, outer leaves removed, washed, dried, torn into bite-size pieces, and chilled

½   cup chopped fresh parsley

½   sweet white onion, sliced thin

½   cup freshly grated Parmesan cheese, plus more for sprinkling on top

Green bell pepper, thinly sliced for garnish (optional)

To make the dressing: In a large salad bowl mash the garlic, salt, and pepper to a paste. Add the mayonnaise, continuing to mash until smooth. Then mix in the lemon juice and the vinegar, if using. Gradually whisk in the olive oil.

Add the romaine and iceberg lettuce, parsley, onion, and the ½ cup of Parmesan. Toss gently. Pile the mixture into shallow salad bowls, sprinkle with a little Parmesan, and serve.

Garnish with bell pepper, if using.

At Joe's, the Armand salad is served at lunch only, and garlic croutons top the dish. In order to keep this within Phase 1, we have omitted the croutons. If you're visiting the famous Joe's, you can ask that the croutons be left off. The stone crabs are great on any phase!

Serves 6

NUTRITION AT A GLANCE
Per serving: 176 calories, 4 g protein, 4 g carbohydrates, 16 g fat, 3 g saturated fats, 238 mg sodium, 6 mg cholesterol, 2 g fiber

Fish Kabobs

2 tablespoons extra-virgin olive oil

2 tablespoons fresh lime juice

1 tablespoon Dijon mustard

1 pound fresh halibut, scrod, swordfish, salmon, or tuna steak, cut 1" thick

½ large red onion, cut lengthwise into quarters

½ green bell pepper, cored, seeded, and cut into 4 wedges

½ red bell pepper, cored, seeded, and cut into 4 wedges

4 cherry tomatoes, stemmed

Combine the oil, juice, and mustard in an 8" x 8" glass baking dish. Stir to blend. Cut the fish into sixteen 1" cubes. Add in one layer to the marinade. Cover and marinate in the refrigerator for 5–10 minutes. Turn the fish cubes to coat evenly and chill 5 minutes longer.

Preheat the broiler. Drain the fish cubes, reserving the marinade. Separate the onion layers slightly. Thread the fish and vegetables onto four skewers, alternating fish cubes with onions, peppers, and tomatoes. Brush the kabobs lightly with the reserved marinade.

Place the skewers on a broiler pan and broil 4" from the heat source, about 3 minutes. Turn the kabobs and brush again with the marinade. Broil for 3–4 minutes longer or until the fish is no longer translucent and the vegetables are tender-crisp.

Serve immediately.

Serves 4

NUTRITION AT A GLANCE

Per serving: 216 calories, 25 g protein, 6 g carbohydrates, 10 g fat, 1 g saturated fats, 158 mg sodium, 36 mg cholesterol, 1 g fiber

Grilled Mahi Mahi

1 pound mahi mahi, fresh or frozen

2 teaspoons olive oil

2 teaspoons lemon juice

¼ teaspoon salt

   Fresh ground pepper to taste

2 cloves garlic, minced

   Capers (optional)

Cut the mahi mahi into 4 serving-size portions. Brush both sides of the fish with the olive oil and lemon juice. Sprinkle with salt and pepper, then rub the garlic on the fish.

To grill, arrange the fish on a grill rack or use a grill basket that has been sprayed with an olive oil cooking spray. Grill over medium-hot coals for 4–6 minutes per ½" of thickness, or until the fish flakes easily when tested with a fork. If the fish is more than 1" thick, gently turn it halfway through grilling.

To broil, arrange the fish on the rack of a broiler pan that has been sprayed with an olive oil cooking spray. Broil 4" from the heat for 4–6 minutes per ½" of thickness, or until the fish flakes easily when tested with a fork. If the fish is more than 1" thick, gently turn it halfway through broiling.

To serve, top the fish with capers, if using.

Serves 4

NUTRITION AT A GLANCE

Per serving: 120 calories, 21 g protein, 1 g carbohydrates, 3 g fat, 1 g saturated fats, 245 mg sodium, 83 mg cholesterol, 0 g fiber

Oven-Roasted Vegetables

1   medium zucchini, cut into bite-size pieces

1   medium summer squash, cut into bite-size pieces

1   medium red bell pepper, cut into bite-size pieces

1   medium yellow bell pepper, cut into bite-size pieces

1   pound fresh asparagus, cut into bite-size pieces

1   red onion

3   tablespoons extra-virgin olive oil

1   teaspoon salt

½   teaspoon freshly ground black pepper

Heat the oven to 450°F. Place the zucchini, squash, peppers, asparagus, and onion in a large roasting pan. Toss with the olive oil, salt, and pepper to mix and coat. Spread in a single layer in the pan. Roast for 30 minutes, stirring occasionally, until the vegetables are lightly browned and tender.

Serves 4

NUTRITION AT A GLANCE

Per serving: 170 calories, 5 g protein,
15 g carbohydrates, 11 g fat, 2 g saturated fats,
586 mg sodium, 0 mg cholesterol, 5 g fiber

Roasted Eggplant and Peppers

1 eggplant, peeled, halved, and sliced

2 red bell peppers, cut in thick strips

1 green bell pepper, cut in thick strips

1 onion, sliced

¼ cup extra-virgin olive oil

Fresh basil (optional)

Preheat the oven to 350°F. Place the eggplant, peppers, and onion in a nonstick baking dish. Drizzle with the oil. Bake in the oven for 20 minutes, basting regularly in its own liquid.

Arrange the vegetables on a serving dish and garnish with fresh basil, if using.

Serves 4

NUTRITION AT A GLANCE

Per serving: 193 calories, 2 g protein,
16 g carbohydrates, 14 g fat, 2 g saturated fats,
5 mg sodium, 0 mg cholesterol, 5 g fiber

Spinach-Stuffed Mushrooms

1 package (10 ounces) frozen chopped spinach

⅛ teaspoon salt

8 large mushrooms

1 tablespoon extra-virgin olive oil

In a medium saucepan, bring ½ cup water to a boil. Add the spinach and salt. Cover, and cook according to package directions. Wash the mushrooms. Remove the stems, trim off the ends, then chop the stems.

Heat the olive oil in a large skillet. Add the chopped mushroom stems. Sauté until golden, about 3 minutes. Remove from the pan. Add the mushroom caps to the skillet and sauté for 4–5 minutes. Remove the mushroom caps to a heatproof serving platter.

Drain the spinach. Stir in the sautéed chopped mushrooms.

Spoon the spinach mixture into the caps and serve immediately or place in the oven on low heat to keep warm.

8 servings

NUTRITION AT A GLANCE

Per serving: 33 calories, 2 g protein,
3 g carbohydrates, 2 g fat, 0 g saturated fats,
74 mg sodium, 0 mg cholesterol, 2 g fiber

Surprise South Beach Mashed "Potatoes"

4 cups cauliflower florets

1 ounce I Can't Believe It's Not Butter! Spray

1 ounce Land O'Lakes Gourmet Fat-Free Half & Half

Pinch salt

Pinch freshly ground black pepper

Steam or microwave the cauliflower until soft. Puree in a food processor, adding the butter spray and the half-and-half to taste. Season with salt and pepper.

Serves 4

NUTRITION AT A GLANCE

Per serving: 81 calories, 2 g protein, 5 g carbohydrates, 6 g fat, 2 g saturated fats, 82 mg sodium, 4 mg cholesterol, 3 g fiber

Stewed Tomatoes and Onions

½ cup chopped green bell pepper

¼ cup thinly sliced celery

1 small onion, chopped

1 clove garlic, minced

3 cups peeled, chopped tomatoes

1 tablespoon red wine vinegar

⅛ teaspoon freshly ground black pepper

Coat a large nonstick skillet with cooking spray. Place over medium–high heat until hot. Add the bell pepper, celery, onion, and garlic. Sauté for 5 minutes or until the vegetables are tender. Add the tomatoes, vinegar, and black pepper.

Bring to a boil. Cover, reduce the heat, and simmer for 15 minutes, stirring occasionally.

Serves 6

NUTRITION AT A GLANCE

Per serving: 29 calories, 1 g protein,
7 g carbohydrates, 0 g fat, 0 g saturated fats,
10 mg sodium, 0 mg cholesterol, 1 g fiber

Broiled Tomatoes

2 large ripe red tomatoes, halved horizontally

Pinch salt (optional)

Pinch freshly ground black pepper (optional)

Place the tomatoes on a broiler pan rack, cut sides facing up. Sprinkle with salt and pepper, if using. Broil for 7–10 minutes, until well-browned.

Serves 2

NUTRITION AT A GLANCE

Per serving: 38 calories, 2 g protein, 8 g carbohydrates, 1 g fat, 0 g saturated fats, 16 mg sodium, 0 mg cholesterol, 2 g fiber

Broiled Tomato with Pesto

3 fresh tomatoes

2 cloves garlic

1 cup chopped fresh basil leaves

2 tablespoons extra-virgin olive oil

¼ cup freshly grated Parmesan cheese

2 tablespoons pine nuts

Cut the tomatoes in half. Combine the garlic, basil, olive oil, Parmesan, and pine nuts in a blender or food processor. Puree until smooth. Spoon the mixture onto the top of each tomato half. Place the tomatoes on a broiler pan and broil about 3" from the heat until lightly browned, about 3–5 minutes.

Serves 6

NUTRITION AT A GLANCE

Per serving: 90 calories, 3 g protein, 4 g carbohydrates, 7 g fat, 2 g saturated fats, 68 mg sodium, 3 mg cholesterol, 1 g fiber

From the Menu of . . .

JOE'S STONE CRAB

11 Washington Avenue, Miami Beach

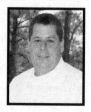

EXECUTIVE CHEF: **ANDRE BIENVENUE**

Joe's Mustard Sauce

1 tablespoon + ½ teaspoon Colman's dry mustard, or more

1 cup mayonnaise

2 teaspoons Worcestershire sauce

1 teaspoon A.1. Steak Sauce

1 tablespoon heavy cream

1 tablespoon milk

Salt

Place the mustard in a mixing bowl or the bowl of an electric mixer. Add the mayonnaise and beat for 1 minute. Add the Worcestershire sauce, steak sauce, cream, milk, and a pinch of salt. Beat until the mixture is well-blended and creamy. If you'd like a little more mustard flavor, whisk in about ½ teaspoon more dry mustard until well-blended. Chill the sauce, covered, until ready to serve.

The stone crabs at Joe's are served cold and already cracked. They come with small metal cups of mustard sauce and melted butter. They are fabulous and great for Phase I if you're visiting Miami Beach!

Makes about 1 cup

NUTRITION AT A GLANCE
Per tablespoon: 109 calories, 0 g protein, 0 g carbohydrates, 12 g fat, 2 g saturated fats, 87 mg sodium, 6 mg cholesterol, 0 g fiber

Edamame Salad

1 bag (16 ounces) frozen shelled edamame (green soybeans)

¼ cup seasoned rice vinegar

1 tablespoon vegetable oil

¼ teaspoon salt

⅛ teaspoon freshly ground black pepper

1 bunch radishes (8 ounces), cut in half and thinly sliced

1 cup loosely packed chopped fresh cilantro leaves

Toss the edamame, vinegar, oil, salt, pepper, radishes, and cilantro together in a large bowl.

Serve chilled or at room temperature.

If edamame is not readily available, you may substitute chick peas.

Serves 4

NUTRITION AT A GLANCE

Per serving: 224 calories, 15 g protein,
18 g carbohydrates, 12 g fat, 1 g saturated fats,
479 mg sodium, 0 mg cholesterol, 6 g fiber

Asian Style Cabbage Salad

½ small head green cabbage

3 scallions, chopped

2 tablespoons dark sesame oil

2 tablespoons rice wine vinegar

2 tablespoons sesame seeds, toasted

Combine the cabbage, scallions, oil, and vinegar. Toss well and chill until ready to serve.

Add the sesame seeds and toss again before serving.

Serves 4

NUTRITION AT A GLANCE

Per serving: 103 calories, 2 g protein,
5 g carbohydrates, 9 g fat, 1 g saturated fats,
15 mg sodium, 0 mg cholesterol, 2 g fiber

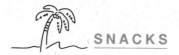 SNACKS

Hummus

1   can (15 ounces) chickpeas

2   tablespoons fresh lemon juice

½   cup tahini (sesame paste)

¼   cup chopped yellow onion

3   cloves garlic, chopped

2   teaspoons extra-virgin olive oil

2   teaspoons ground cumin

⅛   teaspoon ground red pepper

½   teaspoon salt

    Chopped fresh parsley (optional)

Drain the chickpeas, reserving ¼–½ cup of the liquid.

Combine the chickpeas, lemon juice, tahini, onion, garlic, oil, cumin, pepper, and salt in a blender or food processor. Puree until smooth, adding the chickpea liquid if needed to thin the puree.

Refrigerate for 3–4 hours before serving to blend the flavors. Garnish with parsley, if using.

Serves 5

NUTRITION AT A GLANCE

Per serving: 251 calories, 8 g protein,
23 g carbohydrates, 16 g fat, 2 g saturated fats,
447 mg sodium, 0 mg cholesterol, 5 g fiber

Turkey Roll-Ups

4 slices turkey breast

4 medium Boston lettuce leaves

   Cilantro Mayonnaise (see below)

4 scallions

4 red bell pepper strips

Place 1 slice of turkey on a lettuce leaf spread with Cilantro Mayonnaise (see below). Add 1 scallion and 1 pepper strip. Fold into a tight, cigarlike roll.

Ham may be substituted for the turkey. Cilantro Mayonnaise can be used as a dip instead of a spread.

Serves 2

NUTRITION AT A GLANCE

Per serving: 54 calories, 10 g protein, 2 g carbohydrates, 1 g fat, 0 g saturated fats, 604 mg sodium, 17 mg cholesterol, 1 g fiber

Cilantro Mayonnaise

¾ cup reduced-fat mayonnaise

¾ cup loosely packed cilantro leaves

1 tablespoon fresh lime juice

1 teaspoon light soy sauce

1 small clove garlic

Place the mayonnaise, cilantro, lime juice, soy sauce, and garlic in a blender or food processor. Blend until smooth.

Yield ¾ cup

NUTRITION AT A GLANCE

Per tablespoon: 36 calories, 0 g protein, 3 g carbohydrates, 3 g fat, 1 g saturated fats, 104 mg sodium, 4 mg cholesterol, 0 g fiber

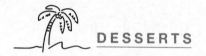 <u>DESSERTS</u>

Lemon Zest Ricotta Crème

½ cup part-skim ricotta cheese

¼ teaspoon grated lemon zest

¼ teaspoon vanilla extract

1 package sugar substitute

Mix together the ricotta, lemon zest, vanilla extract, and sugar substitute in a dessert bowl. Serve chilled.

Serves 1

NUTRITION AT A GLANCE

Per serving: 178 calories, 14 g protein,
7 g carbohydrates, 10 g fat, 6 g saturated fats,
155 mg sodium, 38 mg cholesterol, 0 g fiber

Almond Ricotta Crème

½ cup part-skim ricotta cheese

¼ teaspoon almond extract

1 package sugar substitute

1 teaspoon slivered toasted almonds

Mix together the ricotta, almond extract, and sugar substitute in a dessert bowl. Serve chilled and sprinkled with toasted almonds.

Serves 1

NUTRITION AT A GLANCE

Per serving: 192 calories, 15 g protein,
8 g carbohydrates, 11 g fat, 6 g saturated fats,
155 mg sodium, 38 mg cholesterol, 0 g fiber

Vanilla Ricotta Crème

½ cup part-skim ricotta cheese

¼ teaspoon vanilla extract

1 package sugar substitute

Mix together the ricotta, vanilla extract, and sugar substitute in a dessert bowl. Serve chilled.

Serves 1

NUTRITION AT A GLANCE

Per serving: 178 calories, 14 g protein,
7 g carbohydrates, 10 g fat, 6 g saturated fats,
155 mg sodium, 38 mg cholesterol, 0 g fiber

Mocha Ricotta Crème

½ cup part-skim ricotta cheese

½ teaspoon unsweetened cocoa powder

¼ teaspoon vanilla extract

1 package sugar substitute

Dash espresso powder

5 mini chocolate chips

Mix together the ricotta, cocoa powder, vanilla extract, and sugar substitute in a dessert bowl. Serve chilled with a dusting of espresso powder and sprinkled with the mini chocolate chips.

Serves 1

NUTRITION AT A GLANCE

Per serving: 261 calories, 15 g protein, 17 g carbohydrates, 14 g fat, 9 g saturated fats, 166 mg sodium, 42 mg cholesterol, 0 g fiber

Lime Zest Ricotta Crème

½ cup part-skim ricotta cheese

¼ teaspoon grated lime zest

¼ teaspoon vanilla extract

1 package sugar substitute

Mix together the ricotta, lime zest, vanilla extract, and sugar substitute in a dessert bowl. Serve chilled.

Serves 1

NUTRITION AT A GLANCE

Per serving: 178 calories, 14 g protein, 7 g carbohydrates, 10 g fat, 6 g saturated fats, 155 mg sodium, 38 mg cholesterol, 0 g fiber

PHASE TWO
Meal Plan

We recommend that after 2 weeks of Phase 1, you switch to this more liberal version of the diet. Here's where you begin to gradually reintroduce certain healthy carbs—fruit, whole grain bread, whole grain rice, whole wheat pasta, sweet potatoes—into your diet. The weight loss slows a little during Phase 2, which is why some dieters stay on Phase 1 longer than the 2-week period. If you're confident that you can stick to the stricter plan for another week or two, feel free. But bear in mind that the relatively limited choices on Phase 1 make it a bad choice for a long-term diet. You should stay on Phase 2 until you hit your target weight, at which point you move on to Phase 3. But there will be times during the course of your weight-loss regimen that you will fall off the wagon—maybe you'll overindulge in sweets during a vacation, or around the holidays. Maybe there will be some stressful period that will lead you to put a few pounds back on. When that happens, we suggest that you switch back to Phase 1, just until you lose what you gained and get yourself back on track. That's how we designed the South Beach Diet—the three phases allow enough flexibility to accommodate real life.

Day 1

Breakfast

1 cup fresh strawberries

Oatmeal (½ cup old-fashioned oatmeal mixed with1 cup nonfat milk, cooked on low heat, and sprinkled with cinnamon and 1 Tbsp chopped walnuts)

Decaffeinated coffee or decaffeinated tea with nonfat milk and sugar substitute

Midmorning snack

1 hard-boiled egg

Lunch

Mediterranean Chicken Salad (page 208)

Midafternoon snack

Fresh pear with 1 wedge Laughing Cow Light Cheese

Dinner

Spinach-Stuffed Salmon Fillet (page 224)

Vegetable medley

Tossed salad (mixed greens, cucumbers, green peppers, cherry tomatoes)

Olive oil and vinegar to taste, or 2 Tbsp low-sugar prepared dressing

Dessert

Chocolate-Dipped Strawberries (page 240)

Day 2

Breakfast

Berry smoothie (8 oz non-fat, sugar-free fruit-flavored yogurt, ½ cup berries, ½ cup crushed ice; blend until smooth)

Decaffeinated coffee or decaffeinated tea with nonfat milk and sugar substitute

Midmorning snack

1 hard-boiled egg

Lunch

Lemon Couscous Chicken (page 210)

Tomato and cucumber slices

Midafternoon snack

4 oz non-fat, sugar-free yogurt

Dinner

Meat Loaf (page 221)

Steamed asparagus

Mushrooms sautéed in olive oil

Sliced Bermuda onion and tomato drizzled with olive oil

Dessert

Sliced cantaloupe with 2 Tbsp ricotta cheese

Day 3

Breakfast

1 cup high-fiber cereal (such as Uncle Sam) with ¾ cup nonfat milk

1 cup fresh strawberries

Decaffeinated coffee or decaffeinated tea with nonfat milk and sugar substitute

Midmorning snack

Small Granny Smith apple with 1 Tbsp peanut butter

Lunch

Greek Salad (page 137)

Midafternoon snack

4 oz non-fat, sugar-free yogurt

Dinner

Herb-Marinated Chicken (page 217)

Perfection Salad (page 233)

Steamed julienned zucchini and yellow squash

Dessert

Fresh pear with ricotta cheese and walnuts

Day 4

Breakfast

½ fresh grapefruit

1 slice toasted whole wheat bread topped with 1 ounce sliced reduced-fat Cheddar cheese, broiled until cheese melts

Decaffeinated coffee or decaffeinated tea with nonfat milk and sugar substitute

Midmorning snack

4 oz non-fat, sugar-free yogurt

Lunch

Chef's salad (at least 1 oz each turkey, roast beef, and low-fat cheese on mixed greens)

2 Tbsp Balsamic Vinaigrette (page 148) or low-sugar prepared dressing

Midafternoon snack

Small Granny Smith apple with 1 wedge Laughing Cow Light Cheese

Dinner

Asian Style Chicken Packets with Vegetables (page 219)

Asian Style Cabbage Salad (page 177)

Dessert

Almond Ricotta Crème (page 181)

Day 5

Breakfast

Berry Smoothie (8 oz non-fat, sugar-free fruit-flavored yogurt, ½ cup berries, ½ cup crushed ice; blend until smooth)

Decaffeinated coffee or decaffeinated tea with nonfat milk and sugar substitute

Midmorning snack

1 hard-boiled egg

Lunch

Open-faced roast beef sandwich (3 oz lean roast beef, lettuce, tomato, onion, mustard, 1 slice whole grain bread)

Midafternoon snack

4 oz non-fat, sugar-free yogurt

Dinner

Stir-Fry Chicken and Vegetables (page 215)

Tossed salad (mixed greens, cucumbers, green peppers, cherry tomatoes) Olive oil and vinegar to taste or 2 Tbsp low-sugar prepared dressing

Dessert

½ cup fat-free, sugar-free vanilla pudding with 3–4 sliced strawberries

Day 6

Breakfast

6 oz vegetable juice cocktail

1 poached egg

1 whole wheat English muffin

Decaffeinated coffee or decaffeinated tea with nonfat milk and sugar substitute

Midmorning snack

Small Granny Smith apple with 1 Tbsp peanut butter

Lunch

¾ cup cottage cheese with ¼ cantaloupe, sliced

4 whole wheat crackers

Sugar-free flavored gelatin dessert

Midafternoon snack

Hummus (page 178) with raw vegetables

(May use store-bought hummus)

Dinner

Easy Chicken in Wine Sauce (page 216)

Italian-Style Spaghetti Squash (page 229)

Arugula, spinach, and walnut salad

Olive oil and balsamic vinegar to taste or 2 Tbsp prepared low-sugar dressing

Dessert

Pistachio Bark (page 241)

Day 7

Breakfast

¼ cantaloupe

1 slice toasted whole wheat bread topped with 1 oz sliced reduced-fat Cheddar cheese, broiled until cheese melts

Decaffeinated coffee or decaffeinated tea with nonfat milk and sugar substitute

Midmorning snack

4 oz non-fat, sugar-free yogurt

Lunch

Tomato stuffed with tuna salad (3 oz water-packed tuna, 1 tablespoon chopped celery, 1 tablespoon mayonnaise), served on a bed of salad greens

Midafternoon snack

Baba Ghannouj (page 239) with raw vegetables or wrapped in a lettuce leaf

Dinner

Marinated Flank Steak (page 156)

Green and yellow wax beans with red pepper sautéed in olive oil

Surprise South Beach Mashed "Potatoes" (page 171)

Tossed salad (mixed greens, cucumbers, green peppers, cherry tomatoes)

Olive oil and vinegar to taste or 2 Tbsp low-sugar prepared dressing

Dessert

Sliced cantaloupe with lime wedge

Day 8

Breakfast

Sunrise Parfait (page 202)

Decaffeinated coffee or decaffeinated tea with nonfat milk and sugar substitute

Midmorning snack

1 hard-boiled egg

Lunch

Apple-Walnut Chicken Salad (page 205)

Midafternoon snack

4 oz non-fat, sugar-free yogurt

Dinner

Broiled Sole in Light Cream Sauce (page 225)

Broiled Tomatoes (page 173)

Bibb lettuce salad

Olive oil and balsamic vinegar to taste or 2 Tbsp prepared low-sugar dressing

Dessert

Lemon Zest Ricotta Créme (page 180)

Day 9

Breakfast

Eggs Florentine (1 poached egg served on ½ cup spinach sautéed in olive oil)

Decaffeinated coffee or decaffeinated tea with nonfat milk and sugar substitute

Midmorning snack

Small Granny Smith apple with 1 Tbsp peanut butter

Lunch

Tomato-Basil Couscous Salad (page 209)

Midafternoon snack

4 oz non-fat, sugar-free yogurt

Dinner

Salsa Chicken (page 218)

Tossed salad (mixed greens, cucumbers, green peppers, cherry tomatoes)

2 Tbsp Balsamic Vinaigrette (page 148) or 2 Tbsp prepared low-sugar dressing

Dessert

Chocolate Cups (page 242)

Day 10

Breakfast

Oatmeal Pancake (page 201)

Decaffeinated coffee or decaffeinated tea with nonfat milk and sugar substitute

Midmorning snack

Small Granny Smith apple with 1 Tbsp peanut butter

Lunch

Chicken and Raspberry Spinach Salad (cold chicken breast left over from Day 9) (page 204)

Midafternoon snack

4 oz non-fat, sugar-free yogurt

Dinner

Meat Loaf (page 221)

Italian-Style Spaghetti Squash (page 229)

Dessert

Strawberries with Splenda (or sugar substitute of your choice) or dollop of fat-free frozen whipped topping

Day 11

Breakfast

1 cup fresh strawberries

1 cup high-fiber cereal (such as Uncle Sam) with ¾ cup nonfat milk

Decaffeinated coffee or decaffeinated tea with nonfat milk and sugar substitute

Midmorning snack

1 hard-boiled egg

Lunch

Turkey-tomato pita (3 oz sliced turkey, 3 tomato slices, ½ cup shredded lettuce, 1 tsp Dijon mustard in a whole wheat pita)

Midafternoon snack

4 oz non-fat, sugar-free yogurt

Dinner

Cod en Papillote (page 228)

Bibb lettuce salad

Olive oil and balsamic vinegar to taste or 2 Tbsp prepared low-sugar dressing

Dessert

Baked apple

Day 12

Breakfast

½ grapefruit

1 egg, any style

1 slice 7-grain bread

Low-sugar preserves

Decaffeinated coffee or decaffeinated tea with nonfat milk and sugar substitute

Midmorning snack

1 part-skim mozzarella cheese stick

Lunch

Tomato Soup (page 214)

Chopped sirloin beef patty with 1 slice tomato and 1 slice onion in ½ whole wheat pita

Midafternoon snack

Baba Ghannouj (page 239) with raw vegetables or wrapped in a lettuce leaf

Dinner

Grilled Chicken Salad with Tzatziki Sauce (page 231)

Broiled asparagus with drizzled olive oil

Tossed salad (mixed greens, cucumbers, green peppers, cherry tomatoes)

2 Tbsp Balsamic Vinaigrette (page 148) or 2 Tbsp prepared low-sugar dressing

Dessert

Fresh pear with ricotta cheese and walnuts

Day 13

Breakfast

1 cup blueberries

1 scrambled egg with tomato salsa

Oatmeal (½ cup old-fashioned oatmeal mixed with 1 cup nonfat milk, cooked on low heat, and sprinkled with cinnamon and 1 Tbsp chopped walnuts)

Decaffeinated coffee or decaffeinated tea with nonfat milk and sugar substitute

Midmorning snack

4 oz non-fat, sugar-free yogurt

Lunch

Tuna salad (3 oz water-packed tuna, 1 tablespoon chopped celery, 1 tablespoon mayonnaise), 3 slices tomato, 3 slices onion in a whole wheat pita

Midafternoon snack

1 part-skim mozzarella cheese stick

Dinner

Pan-Roasted Steak and Onions (page 220)

South Beach Salad (page 232)

Steamed broccoli

Dessert

Chocolate-Dipped Strawberries (page 240)

Day 14

Breakfast

6 oz vegetable juice cocktail

Baked eggs in Canadian bacon cups

1 slice 7-grain bread, toasted

Decaffeinated coffee or decaffeinated tea with nonfat milk and sugar substitute

Midmorning snack

4 oz non-fat, sugar-free yogurt

Lunch

Portobello Pizza (page 211)

Midafternoon snack

Small Granny Smith apple with 1 wedge Laughing Cow Light Cheese

Dinner

Grilled salmon

Couscous

White Asparagus Salad (page 236)

Dessert

Fresh Strawberries with Lime Zest Ricotta Crème (page 182)

FOODS YOU CAN
REINTRODUCE TO YOUR DIET

FRUIT
Apples
Apricots
   dried
   fresh
Bananas (medium)
Blueberries
Cantaloupe
Cherries
Grapefruit
Grapes
Kiwi
Mangoes
Oranges
Peaches
Pears
Plums
Strawberries

DAIRY
Yogurt, non-fat flavored, artificially
sweetened

STARCHES (USE SPARINGLY)
Bagels, small, whole grain
Bread
   multigrain
   oat and bran
   rye
   whole wheat
Cereal
   Fiber One
   Kellogg's Extra-Fiber All Bran
   Oatmeal (not instant)
   Other high-fiber
   Uncle Sam

Muffins, bran
   sugar-free (no raisins)
Pasta, whole wheat
Peas, green
Pita
   stone-ground
   whole wheat
Popcorn
Potato, small, sweet
Rice
   brown
   wild

VEGETABLES AND LEGUMES
Barley
Beans, pinto
Black-eyed peas
Carrots

MISCELLANEOUS
Chocolate (sparingly)
   bittersweet
   semisweet
Pudding, fat-free, sugar-free
Wine, red or white

FOODS TO AVOID OR EAT RARELY

STARCHES AND BREADS

Bagel, refined wheat

Bread

  refined wheat

  white

Cookies

Cornflakes

Matzo

Pasta, white flour

Potatoes

  baked, white

  instant

Rice cakes

Rice, white

Rolls, dinner

VEGETABLES

Beets

Corn

Potatoes

FRUIT

Canned fruit, juice packed

Fruit juice

Pineapple

Raisins

Watermelon

MISCELLANEOUS

Honey

Ice cream

Jam

PHASE TWO

Recipes

Now that you've resolved your insulin resistance and lost a dozen or so pounds, you're ready to settle into a long-term weight-loss program. Phase 2 begins to gradually reintroduce carbohydrates into your diet, starting with low–glycemic index ones such as oatmeal and couscous. The recipes herein still don't recommend even good high-glycemic carbohydrates, such as sweet potatoes, whole wheat pasta, or whole grain bread or rice; the diet's flexibility allows you to begin adding these unprocessed carbs into your meals as you see fit. In this phase the desserts also become more liberal, allowing, for instance, Chocolate-Dipped Strawberries.

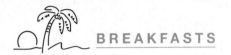 **BREAKFASTS**

Oatmeal Pancake

½ cup old-fashioned oatmeal

¼ cup low-fat cottage cheese (or tofu)

4 egg whites

1 teaspoon vanilla extract

¼ teaspoon cinnamon

¼ teaspoon nutmeg

Process the oatmeal, cottage cheese, egg whites, vanilla extract, cinnamon, and nutmeg in a blender until smooth.

Spray a nonstick skillet with cooking spray. Add the batter and cook over medium heat until both sides are lightly browned.

You can top the pancake with a low-sugar syrup of your choice.

Serves 1

NUTRITION AT A GLANCE

Per serving: 288 calories, 28 g protein,
32 g carbohydrates, 4 g fat, 1 g saturated fats,
451 mg sodium, 5 mg cholesterol, 5 g fiber

Sunrise Parfait

1   cup sliced strawberries

1   cup non-fat, sugar-free vanilla yogurt

½   cup Uncle Sam cereal

Layer the strawberries, yogurt, and cereal in 2 stemmed dessert glasses.

Serves 2

NUTRITION AT A GLANCE

Per serving: 185 calories, 8 g protein,
37 g carbohydrates, 1 g fat, 0 g saturated fats,
102 mg sodium, 3 mg cholesterol, 6 g fiber

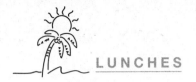

LUNCHES

Poached Salmon Spinach Salad

- 2 tablespoons extra-virgin olive oil
- ½ pound cleaned fresh spinach
- ¼ teaspoon salt
- ⅛ teaspoon freshly ground black pepper
- ½ cup chopped yellow onion
- 3 fresh tomatoes (about 1¼ pounds), peeled, seeded, and cut into ½" pieces

  Poached salmon left over from Poached Salmon with Cucumber-Dill Sauce (page 161)

- 1 tablespoon coarsely chopped flat-leaf parsley (optional)

In a skillet, heat 1 tablespoon of the oil over medium heat. When hot, sauté the spinach for 1½ minutes. Mix in the salt and pepper and divide the spinach among 4 plates.

Heat the remaining tablespoon of oil in the skillet. Sauté the onion and tomatoes over medium heat until the onion is tender, about 5–6 minutes.

Arrange the salmon on the spinach and top with the tomatoes and onion. Garnish with parsley, if using.

Serves 4

NUTRITION AT A GLANCE

Per serving: 98 calories, 2 g protein,
9 g carbohydrates, 7 g fat, 1 g saturated fats,
162 mg sodium, 0 mg cholesterol, 2 g fiber

Chicken and Raspberry Spinach Salad

¼ cup raspberry vinegar or white wine vinegar

5 tablespoons extra-virgin olive oil

1 teaspoon honey

½ teaspoon finely shredded orange peel

⅛ teaspoon salt

¼ teaspoon freshly ground black pepper

4 boneless, skinless chicken breast halves (about 12 ounces total)

8–10 cups torn spinach or torn mixed greens

1 cup fresh raspberries

1 papaya, peeled, seeded, and sliced

In a screw-top jar, combine the vinegar, 4 tablespoons of the oil, the honey, orange peel, salt, and pepper. Cover and shake well. Chill the dressing until serving time.

In a medium skillet, cook the chicken in the remaining 1 tablespoon of oil over medium heat for 8–10 minutes or until the chicken is tender and no longer pink. Turn the chicken often to brown evenly. Remove the chicken from the skillet. Cut into thin, bite-size strips.

In a large bowl, toss together the warm chicken strips and the spinach or mixed greens. Shake the dressing well. Add the dressing and raspberries to the chicken mixture. Toss lightly to coat well.

Divide the chicken mixture among 4 salad plates. Arrange the papaya slices on each plate.

You may substitute 2 medium nectarines, pitted and sliced; or 2 peaches, peeled, pitted, and sliced for the papaya.

Serves 4

NUTRITION AT A GLANCE

Per serving: 320 calories, 22 g protein,
16 g carbohydrates, 19 g fat, 3 g saturated fats,
199 mg sodium, 49 mg cholesterol, 5 g fiber

Apple-Walnut Chicken Salad

5 ounces cooked chicken breast, cut into ½"–¾" chunks

½ cup chopped celery

¾ cup chopped apple

2 ounces chopped walnuts

1 tablespoon raisins

⅓ cup prepared low-sugar Italian dressing

Bibb lettuce

In a medium bowl, gently stir together the chicken, celery, apple, walnuts, and raisins. Pour the dressing over the mixture and toss gently to coat.

Serve on a bed of Bibb lettuce.

Serves 2

NUTRITION AT A GLANCE

Per serving: 444 calories, 27 g protein, 33 g carbohydrates, 25 g fat, 3 g saturated fats, 391 mg sodium, 63 mg cholesterol, 8 g fiber

From the Menu of ...

BLUE DOOR AT DELANO

1685 Collins Avenue, Miami Beach

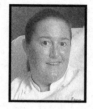

EXECUTIVE CHEF: ELIZABETH BARLOW

LOCATED IN THE DELANO HOTEL, ONE OF MIAMI BEACH'S HOTTEST DESTINATION RESORTS, BLUE DOOR WAS NAMED ONE OF AMERICA'S BEST NEW RESTAURANTS FOR 1998 BY ESQUIRE MAGAZINE. IN A CHIC, ART DECO SETTING, CONSULTING CHEF CLAUDE TROISGROS HAS TEAMED WITH CHEF ELIZABETH BARLOW TO PRODUCE MODERN, FRENCH–BASED CUISINE WITH A TROPICAL INFLUENCE.

Veal Moutarde 4 Pax

4   medium shallots, minced

2   cloves garlic, minced

3   teaspoons butter

2   teaspoons Dijon mustard

2   teaspoons balsamic vinegar

4   cups veal stock or beef bouillon

4   small vine-ripened tomatoes, peeled, seeded, and cut into medium dice

1   ounce mustard seed

Salt

Freshly ground black pepper

4   veal chops (10 ounces), frenched*

¼   cup olive oil

3   teaspoons butter

4   sprigs fresh rosemary, fried for 10 seconds

4   cloves garlic, roasted

Sauté half of the the shallots and the garlic on medium heat in 1 teaspoon butter until translucent, about 20 to 30 seconds.

Add the mustard and vinegar and cook until the vinegar is almost evaporated, about 1 minute.

Add the veal stock or beef bouillon and reduce by half, to about 2 cups.

Sauté the tomatoes in 2 teaspoons of butter with the remaining shallots for about 1½ minutes. Add the mustard seed.

Strain the reduced veal stock through a sieve and add to the sautéed tomatoes. Add salt and pepper to taste.

Season the veal chops with salt and pepper. Pan sear the chops in the oil for 1½ minutes on each side or until a golden brown crust appears. Place in the oven for 8–12 minutes at 350°F or until desired doneness. Remove from the oven and let rest for 3–4 minutes.

To serve, place a veal chop in the center of a shallow bowl. Pour 2 ounces of sauce around it and garnish with a fried rosemary sprig and a roasted garlic clove.

To french your veal chops, cut off the meat along the bone.

Serves 4

NUTRITION AT A GLANCE
Per serving: 340 calories, 19 g protein, 13 g carbohydrates, 24 g fat, 5 g saturated fats, 958 mg sodium, 56 mg cholesterol, 2 g fiber

Mediterranean Chicken Salad

Dressing

- ½ cup low-sugar prepared Italian dressing
- 1 tablespoon cayenne pepper sauce
- ½ tablespoon dried mint leaves
- ¼ tablespoon mustard powder

Salad

- 1 pound boneless, skinless chicken breast
- 2 tablespoons extra-virgin olive oil
- 2 cups prepared bulgur wheat
- 1½ cups diced cucumbers
- 1½ cups diced tomatoes
- 1 cup minced green onion
- ½ cup chopped fresh parsley

  Romaine lettuce leaves

To make the dressing: Whisk together the Italian dressing, pepper sauce, mint, and mustard powder in a small bowl. Cover and chill until ready to use.

To make the salad: In a medium skillet, cook the chicken in the oil over medium heat for 8–10 minutes or until the chicken is tender and no longer pink. Turn often to brown evenly. Remove the chicken from the skillet. Cut into thin, bite-size cubes. Allow the chicken to cool, then refrigerate until fully chilled.

Combine the chicken with the bulgur, cucumbers, tomatoes, onion, and parsley in a bowl. Serve over the lettuce and drizzle with the dressing.

Serves 6

NUTRITION AT A GLANCE

Per serving: 220 calories, 20 g protein, 18 g carbohydrates, 8 g fat, 1 g saturated fats, 279 mg sodium, 45 mg cholesterol, 4 g fiber

Tomato-Basil Couscous Salad

¾ cup cooked couscous

1 tomato, chopped

⅓ cup canned chickpeas, drained and rinsed

2 scallions, chopped

1 teaspoon extra-virgin olive oil

1 tablespoon fresh lemon juice

1 tablespoon chopped fresh basil

Lettuce

Combine the couscous, tomato, chickpeas, scallions, oil, lemon juice, and basil in a bowl.

Toss, and serve on a bed of lettuce.

Serves 1

NUTRITION AT A GLANCE

Per serving: 43 calories, 2 g protein, 7 g carbohydrates, 1 g fat, 0 g saturated fats, 0 mg sodium, 0 mg cholesterol, 1 g fiber

Lemon Couscous Chicken

1¼ cups water

1 tablespoon extra-virgin olive oil

2 cups broccoli florets

1 package Near East Roasted Garlic & Olive Oil Couscous mix

1½ cups chopped cooked chicken

   Juice of 1 lemon (about 3 tablespoons)

¼ teaspoon lemon peel

In a large skillet, bring the water, oil, broccoli, and contents of the spice sack from the couscous mix to a boil. Stir in the couscous, chicken, lemon juice, and lemon peel. Remove from the heat. Cover and let stand for 5 minutes. Fluff lightly with a fork.

Chill well and serve cold.

Serves 4

NUTRITION AT A GLANCE

Per serving: 311 calories, 24 g protein, 39 g carbohydrates, 7 g fat, 1 g saturated fats, 476 mg sodium, 45 mg cholesterol, 3 g fiber

Portobello Pizza

1   teaspoon extra-virgin olive oil

1   clove garlic, diced

1   package (6 ounces) portobello mushroom caps, cleaned

     Pinch salt

     Pinch freshly ground black pepper

12   ounces mozzarella cheese, sliced or shredded

10   fresh basil leaves

2   fresh tomatoes, sliced, roasted, or grilled

     Oregano leaves (optional)

Preheat the oven to 450°F. Combine the oil and garlic in a small bowl and rub the mushroom caps on all sides with the mixture. Place the caps, top side down, in a circle on an oiled baking sheet. Season with the salt and pepper. Arrange the cheese, basil, and tomato slices alternately in a circle on top of the mushrooms. Sprinkle with the oregano, if using.

Bake at 450°F until the cheese melts, about 3 minutes.

Serves 2

NUTRITION AT A GLANCE

Per serving: 549 calories, 36 g protein,
14 g carbohydrates, 40 g fat, 23 g saturated fats,
651 mg sodium, 133 mg cholesterol, 3 g fiber

From the Menu of . . .

RUMI SUPPER CLUB

330 Lincoln Road, Miami Beach

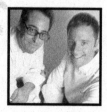

EXECUTIVE CHEFS: SCOTT FREDEL and J. D. HARRIS

WITH AN INNOVATIVE MENU AND A GORGEOUS SETTING, RUMI IS A DESTINATION WHERE FINE DINING TURNS TO DANCING AS THE EVENING DRAWS LATE. SERVING MODERN FLORIDA CARIBBEAN CUISINE, RUMI'S KITCHEN DOES NOT HAVE A FREEZER, AS THE FRESH CATCH IS BROUGHT IN DAILY.

Rumi Chopped Salad with Lemon Vinaigrette

Salad

- 1 beet
- 2 ounces sherry vinegar
- 1 red bell pepper
- 1 ounce pecans
- 1 ounce kalamata olives
- 6 basil leaves
- 1 shallot

Vinaigrette

2 ounces lemon juice

Salt

White pepper

1 egg

1 teaspoon Dijon mustard

3 ounces olive oil

3 ounces canola oil

1 head Belgian endive, thinly sliced

1 ounce frisée leaves

1 orange, peeled and sectioned

To make the salad: Roast the beet until tender and dice. Place the excess beet juice in sherry vinegar and cook to make a beet marinade.

Strain the beet marinade and cover the diced beets with it. Roast the pepper and dice. Roast the pecans and chop them, saving some whole for garnish. Sliver the olives, slice the basil leaves into strips, and chop the shallot finely.

To make the vinaigrette: Place the lemon juice, salt, pepper, egg, and mustard in a blender and mix. Add the oils slowly to create an emulsion.

Mix the endive, frisée, orange, bell pepper, pecans, olives, basil, shallots, and vinaigrette. Place a mound of diced beets (with juice) onto a plate and top with a mound of dressed salad. Garnish with a whole pecan.

Since eggs are unpasteurized, you may want to substitute a liquid, pasteurized egg product (like Egg Beaters). One-quarter cup of liquid egg substitute is the equivalent of 1 whole egg.

Serves 6

NUTRITION AT A GLANCE
Per serving: 338 calories, 2 g protein, 9 g carbohydrates, 33 g fat, 4 g saturated fats, 120 mg sodium, 35 mg cholesterol, 3 g fiber

Tomato Soup

1 small onion, chopped

¼ cup sliced mushrooms

3 ounces diced ham

¼ teaspoon extra-virgin olive oil

1 clove garlic, minced

⅛ teaspoon sweet paprika

   Dash allspice

1 can (14.5 ounces) fat-free chicken broth

1 can (15 ounces) chickpeas

3 whole tomatoes, peeled

Mix the onion, mushrooms, ham, oil, garlic, paprika, and allspice in a large pot. Cook for 1 minute. Add the chicken broth, chickpeas, and tomatoes. Cover and simmer for 15 minutes.

Puree the soup in a blender and serve.

Serves 2

NUTRITION AT A GLANCE

Per serving: 404 calories, 29 g protein,
58 g carbohydrates, 7 g fat, 2 g saturated fats,
1,341 mg sodium, 25 mg cholesterol, 12 g fiber

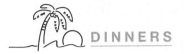

DINNERS

Stir-Fry Chicken and Vegetables

3 tablespoons canola oil

½ pound cooked chicken breast, cut diagonally into ⅛" thick slices

1 package (10 ounces) frozen vegetables containing broccoli, green beans, red bell peppers, and mushrooms

2 tablespoons water

2 tablespoons soy sauce

1 package (10 ounces) fresh spinach

Heat a large, heavy skillet or wok over high heat until water sizzles when dropped onto the metal. Add 1½ tablespoons of the oil and tilt the pan gently in all directions until the oil has coated the surface. When the oil is hot (not to the point of smoking), add the chicken breast slices and stir-fry for 2 minutes. Remove the chicken to a bowl.

Add the remaining oil to the skillet. When hot, add the frozen vegetable mix and stir-fry for about 4 minutes, until the larger pieces are cooked through. Return the chicken to the skillet, add the water and soy sauce, and stir-fry for an additional 2 minutes. Add the spinach. Cover the pan and steam over medium heat for 2 minutes. Using tongs, turn the spinach once so that it heats evenly; cover and steam for an additional 2 minutes.

Remove the chicken and vegetables with a slotted spoon. Spoon the liquid into small bowls and serve as a gravy or dip.

Serves 4

NUTRITION AT A GLANCE

Per serving: 232 calories, 23 g protein,
7 g carbohydrates, 13 g fat, 2 g saturated fats,
616 mg sodium, 48 mg cholesterol, 4 g fiber

Easy Chicken in Wine Sauce

4 tablespoons extra-virgin olive oil

1 clove garlic, crushed

3 boneless, skinless chicken breast halves, cut into strips

⅛ teaspoon salt

¼ teaspoon coarsely ground black pepper

½ cup dry white wine

3 medium tomatoes, sliced

In a medium skillet, heat the oil and garlic over medium heat. Sprinkle the chicken with the salt and pepper, then add to the skillet and cook for 7–10 minutes. Add the white wine and cook for an additional 2 minutes.

Remove the chicken to a platter. Sauté the tomatoes in the skillet until tender. Place the tomatoes over the chicken and cover with the pan drippings.

Serves 4

NUTRITION AT A GLANCE

Per serving: 190 calories, 6 g protein,
5 g carbohydrates, 15 g fat, 2 g saturated fats,
117 mg sodium, 12 mg cholesterol, 1 g fiber

Herb-Marinated Chicken

6 boneless, skinless chicken breast halves

½ cup white wine

2 tablespoons extra-virgin olive or canola oil

1 tablespoon white vinegar

2 teaspoons dried crushed basil

1 teaspoon dried crushed oregano or tarragon

½ teaspoon onion powder

2 cloves garlic, minced

Set a heavy zip-top food-storage bag in a large mixing bowl and place the chicken in the bag. Add the wine, oil, vinegar, basil, oregano or tarragon, onion powder, and garlic. Close the bag and turn it to coat the chicken well. Marinate for 5–24 hours in the refrigerator, turning occasionally.

Drain the chicken, reserving the marinade. Place the chicken on an unheated rack in a broiler pan. Brush with the marinade. Broil 4"–5" from the heat for about 20 minutes or until lightly browned, brushing often with the marinade. Turn the chicken and broil for 5–15 minutes more, until the chicken is tender and no longer pink.

Serves 6

NUTRITION AT A GLANCE

Per serving: 185 calories, 26 g protein,
1 g carbohydrates, 6 g fat, 1 g saturated fats,
75 mg sodium, 66 mg cholesterol, 0 g fiber

Salsa Chicken

8 cups finely shredded iceberg lettuce

3 tablespoons chili powder

1 teaspoon ground cumin

1 pound boneless, skinless chicken breast, cut into 1" pieces

2 large egg whites

2 tablespoons extra-virgin olive oil

8 ounces chunky tomato salsa

½ cup fat-free sour cream

Cilantro sprigs (optional)

Divide the lettuce among 4 individual plates, cover and set aside. In a large bowl, combine the chili powder and cumin. Add the chicken, turning to coat. Lift the chicken from the bowl, shaking off the excess coating. Dip the chicken into the egg whites, then coat again with the remaining dry mixture.

Heat the oil in a wide nonstick frying pan or wok over medium heat. When the oil is hot, add the chicken and stir-fry gently until no longer pink in the center. Cut to test (5–7 minutes). Remove the chicken from the pan and keep warm. Pour the salsa into the pan; reduce the heat to medium and cook, stirring, until the salsa is heated through and slightly thickened.

Arrange the chicken over the lettuce; top with the salsa and sour cream. Garnish with cilantro sprigs, if using.

Serves 4

NUTRITION AT A GLANCE

Per serving: 266 calories, 32 g protein,
12 g carbohydrates, 10 g fat, 2 g saturated fats,
457 mg sodium, 66 mg cholesterol, 5 g fiber

Asian-Style Chicken Packets with Vegetables

⅓ cup dry sherry or vermouth

3 tablespoons reduced-sodium soy sauce

2 teaspoons sesame oil

¼ cup finely chopped green onions

1 teaspoon freshly grated ginger

1 teaspoon finely chopped garlic

4 boneless, skinless chicken breast halves, cut into ½" strips

1 red bell pepper, sliced

1 package (10 ounces) snow peas

1 package (10 ounces) broccoli florets

1 can (5 ounces) water chestnuts

Preheat the oven to 450°F or the grill to medium–high. Mix the sherry or vermouth, soy sauce, oil, onions, ginger, and garlic in a small bowl. Add the chicken, pepper, peas, broccoli, and water chestnuts to the mixture and toss until evenly coated.

Center ¼ of the chicken mixture on each of four 12" x 18" sheets of heavy-duty aluminum foil. Bring up the foil sides; double-fold the tops and ends to seal the packets. Bake for 15–18 minutes on a baking sheet in the oven or grill for 12–14 minutes in a covered grill.

Serves 4

NUTRITION AT A GLANCE

Per serving: 244 calories, 32 g protein,
16 g carbohydrates, 4 g fat, 1 g saturated fats,
855 mg sodium, 66 mg cholesterol, 7 g fiber

Pan-Roasted Steak and Onions

1 tablespoon extra-virgin olive oil

2 tablespoons balsamic vinegar

1 tablespoon Worcestershire sauce

1 tablespoon Dijon mustard

2 cloves garlic, minced

1 pound flank steak

1 tablespoon cracked black pepper

½ teaspoon salt

1 cup fat-free chicken broth

1 medium onion, cut into ¼" thick rings

In a large nonaluminum baking dish, combine the oil, vinegar, Worcestershire sauce, mustard, and garlic. Add the steak; turn to coat. Cover; refrigerate for 30 minutes or overnight, turning once.

Coat a nonstick skillet with cooking spray. Place over medium–high heat. Sprinkle the steak with the pepper and salt. Brown for 2 minutes per side. Add ½ cup of the broth; cook, turning once, for 5–6 minutes per side (for medium-rare). Remove the steak from the skillet; cover the steak loosely to keep it warm. Reduce the heat to medium. Add the onion slices to the skillet and cook until golden brown, about 4–5 minutes per side. Add the remaining broth as needed to prevent the onions from sticking.

Thinly slice the steak across the grain; serve with the onions.

Serves 4

NUTRITION AT A GLANCE

Per serving: 239 calories, 24 g protein, 7 g carbohydrates, 12 g fat, 4 g saturated fats, 580 mg sodium, 55 mg cholesterol, 1 g fiber

Meat Loaf

1   can (6 ounces) no-salt-added tomato paste

½   cup dry red wine

½   cup water

1   clove garlic, minced

½   teaspoon dried basil leaves

¼   teaspoon dried oregano leaves

¼   teaspoon salt

16   ounces ground turkey breast

1   cup oatmeal

¼   cup liquid egg substitute

½   cup shredded zucchini

Preheat the oven to 350°F. Combine the tomato paste, wine, water, garlic, basil, oregano, and salt in a small saucepan. Bring to a boil, then reduce the heat to low. Simmer, uncovered, for 15 minutes. Set aside.

Combine the turkey, oatmeal, egg substitute, zucchini, and ½ cup of the tomato mixture in a large bowl. Mix well. Shape into a loaf and place into an ungreased 8" x 4" loaf pan. Bake for 45 minutes. Discard any drippings. Pour ½ cup of the remaining tomato mixture over the top of the loaf. Bake for an additional 15 minutes.

Place on a serving platter. Cool for 10 minutes before slicing. Serve the remaining tomato sauce on the side.

Serves 8

NUTRITION AT A GLANCE

Per serving: 188 calories, 12 g protein,
12 g carbohydrates, 10 g fat, 3 g saturated fats,
244 mg sodium, 39 mg cholesterol, 2 g fiber

From the Menu of ...

TUSCAN STEAK

431 Washington Avenue, Miami Beach

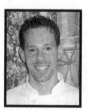

CHEF: **MICHAEL WAGNER**

Grilled Yellowfin Tuna
with a White Bean and Oregano Salad

6	ounces sushi-grade yellowfin tuna
	Salt
	Cracked black pepper
¼	teaspoon crushed garlic
	Juice of half a lemon
2	ounces olive oil
¼	cup water
1	teaspoon fresh basil, chopped
½	tablespoon dried oregano
12	ounces cooked white beans
1	teaspoon parsley, chopped

Season the tuna with the salt and pepper and grill each side for 30–45 seconds. Set aside to cool.

Mix the garlic, lemon juice, olive oil, water, basil, oregano, and beans in a cold mixing bowl and let marinate for 3 hours in the refrigerator.

To serve, bring the salad to room temperature and place it in the middle of a shallow bowl. Slice the tuna thinly, and lay it on top of the bean mixture. Garnish the plate with the chopped parsley.

Serves 4

NUTRITION AT A GLANCE
Per serving: 299 calories, 18 g protein, 23 g carbohydrates, 15 g fat, 2 g saturated fats, 19 mg sodium, 19 mg cholesterol, 10 g fiber

Spinach-Stuffed Salmon Fillets

4 salmon fillets (about 5 ounces each)

Pinch salt

Pinch freshly ground black pepper

1 package (10 ounces) baby spinach, coarsely chopped

2 tablespoons prepared pesto

1 tablespoon chopped dry-packed sun-dried tomatoes

1 tablespoon pine nuts

Heat the oven to 400°F. Make a slit two-thirds of the way through the center of each fillet making sure not to cut all the way through. Season each fillet with the salt and pepper. In a bowl, combine the spinach, pesto, tomatoes, and pine nuts. Spoon ⅓ cup of the mixture into each slit.

Arrange the fillets on a broiler pan coated with cooking spray. Roast for 8–10 minutes or until the spinach mixture is heated through.

Serves 4

NUTRITION AT A GLANCE

Per serving: 329 calories, 32 g protein,
4 g carbohydrates, 20 g fat, 4 g saturated fats,
213 mg sodium, 86 mg cholesterol, 3 g fiber

Broiled Sole in Light Cream Sauce

3 tablespoons I Can't Believe It's Not Butter! spread or spray

1 cup Lea & Perrins White Wine Worcestershire Sauce

¼ cup fat-free half-and-half

4 sole fillets

Place the spread or spray in a medium saucepan. Whisk in the Worcestershire sauce, bring it to a boil and reduce the sauce slightly. Stir in the half-and-half and keep warm.

Meanwhile, preheat the broiler and place the fish on an unheated rack in a broiler pan. Broil 4"–6" from the heat and cook for 2–6 minutes or until it flakes easily. Remove the fish to a serving platter and spoon the sauce over the fish.

Serves 4

NUTRITION AT A GLANCE

Per serving: 262 calories, 27 g protein, 12 g carbohydrates, 11 g fat, 3 g saturated fats, 860 mg sodium, 76 mg cholesterol, 0 g fiber

JOE'S STONE CRAB

11 Washington Avenue, Miami Beach

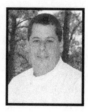

EXECUTIVE CHEF: **ANDRE BIENVENUE**

Shrimp Louis

Shrimp

¾ pound baby or medium-size shrimp

Salt

Juice of 1 small lime

Lettuce leaves

1 cup canned garbanzo beans, drained

1 large ripe tomato, cored and sliced

2 eggs, hard-cooked

2 lemons, cut in half crosswise

4 ripe black olives

4 thin round slices green bell pepper

Louis Dressing:

½ cup mayonnaise

2 tablespoons chili sauce

1   tablespoon grated onion

1   tablespoon chopped fresh parsley

   Salt

   Pepper

1   tablespoon heavy cream, plus extra to reduce thickness

¼   teaspoon Worcestershire sauce, or more

   Several drops Tabasco sauce

To make the shrimp: Drop the shrimp into boiling water flavored with a little salt and lime juice. Cook until just pink, usually 1 to 2 minutes. Drain and cool slightly; shell and devein. Place in a bowl; cover with plastic wrap and chill.

Arrange lettuce leaves to cover two large dinner plates (at Joe's, this is made on large oval plates). Place a mound of shrimp on one side and a mound of garbanzo beans on the other. Place tomato slices in the four "corners" of the plate. Cut the eggs lengthwise in quarters and place a quarter next to each tomato slice. Place a lemon half at the end of each plate and 2 olives at the top and bottom. Place the green pepper rings at the edges. Cover and chill if not serving immediately.

To make the Louis dressing: Combine the mayonnaise, chili sauce, grated onion, parsley, salt, black pepper, cream, Worcestershire sauce, and Tabasco sauce. Stir until blended. Chill, covered, until serving time. If too thick, stir in a little more cream. Serve the dressing in a small sauce-boat beside the shrimp.

This is a good-looking plate. The Louis dressing can be used for other cold seafood, too. Louis dressing contains a large amount of mayonnaise but is not a problem if used as a dip. Don't eat it like soup!

Serves 2

NUTRITION AT A GLANCE
Per serving: 867 calories, 46 g protein, 40 g carbohydrates, 58 g fat, 10 g saturated fats, 1,493 mg sodium, 501 mg cholesterol, 7 g fiber

Cod en Papillote

2 cod steaks, 1" thick (about 1⅓ pounds)

2 tablespoons lemon juice

1 cup thinly sliced mushrooms

½ small zucchini, julienned

½ small red bell pepper, julienned

½ small onion, thinly sliced

2 tablespoons I Can't Believe It's Not Butter! spread or spray

¼ teaspoon dried tarragon leaves

   Pinch freshly ground black pepper

Cut two 2-foot lengths of parchment paper and fold each in half to make a 1-foot square. Place 1 cod steak slightly below the middle of each square of paper. Over each steak, sprinkle half of the lemon juice, mushrooms, zucchini, bell pepper, and onion. Top each with half the butter. Fold the parchment over the fish and crimp the edges together tightly. Place the packets side by side in a microwaveable 13" x 9" x 2" baking dish. Microwave on high for 6 minutes, rotating the dish a half turn after 3 minutes.

To serve, cut an X in the top of each packet with scissors and tear to open.

Serves 2

NUTRITION AT A GLANCE

Per serving: 370 calories, 56 g protein,
7 g carbohydrates, 12 g fat, 2 g saturated fats,
260 mg sodium, 130 mg cholesterol, 2 g fiber

Italian-Style Spaghetti Squash

2 pounds spaghetti squash, halved lengthwise and seeded

2 tablespoons olive oil

1 medium red onion, thinly sliced

1 zucchini (8 ounces), cut into ½" dice

4 medium tomatoes, diced

¼ teaspoon salt

¼ teaspoon coarsely ground pepper

½ cup reduced-fat grated Parmesan cheese (optional)

1 small lemon, sliced

Place the squash halves, cut sides down, in a glass baking dish. Add ¼ cup water and cover with plastic wrap. Microwave on high for 8–10 minutes until tender; cool slightly.

Meanwhile, in a large skillet, heat 1 tablespoon of the oil. Add the onion and cook over medium–high heat for 3 minutes until the onion is translucent. Add the zucchini and cook for 4–5 minutes until the zucchini begins to brown. Add the tomatoes, salt, and pepper. Reduce the heat; simmer gently for 10 minutes.

Using a fork, scrape the squash strands into a bowl. Toss with the remaining tablespoon of oil. Mound the squash in the center of 4 pasta bowls and spoon the vegetable mixture around the squash. Drizzle with more oil, if desired, and garnish with Parmesan cheese, if using. Add the lemon slices.

Serves 4

NUTRITION AT A GLANCE

Per serving: 190 calories, 5 g protein,
28 g carbohydrates, 9 g fat, 1 g saturated fats,
199 mg sodium, 0 mg cholesterol, 6 g fiber

Baked Tomatoes with Basil and Parmesan

3 large vine-ripened tomatoes (about 1½ pounds), cut in half

¼ cup minced fresh herbs (basil, parsley, marjoram)

½ cup dry grated bread crumbs

½ cup shredded Parmesan or Asiago cheese

2 garlic cloves, finely minced

   Pinch salt

   Pinch freshly ground black pepper

3 tablespoons extra-virgin olive oil

Preheat the oven to 350°F. Put the tomatoes in a nonstick baking dish, cut sides up. Combine the herbs, bread crumbs, cheese, garlic, salt, pepper, and oil in a small bowl. Sprinkle each tomato with an equal portion of the mixture.

Bake for 30 minutes or until crusty. Tomatoes will be soft yet hold their shape.

Serves 6

NUTRITION AT A GLANCE

Per serving: 132 calories, 4 g protein,
9 g carbohydrates, 9 g fat, 2 g saturated fats,
161 mg sodium, 5 mg cholesterol, 1 g fiber

Grilled Chicken Salad with Tzatziki Sauce

Chicken

- 1 ounce extra-virgin olive oil
- 2 teaspoons fresh lemon juice
- 1 teaspoon oregano
- ¼ teaspoon kosher salt
- 1 teaspoon cracked black pepper
- 4 boneless, skinless chicken breast halves

Tzatziki Sauce

- 1 cup non-fat plain yogurt
- ⅔ cup peeled, seeded, and diced cucumbers
- ¾ teaspoon minced garlic
- ⅔ ounce extra-virgin olive oil
- ⅔ ounce white vinegar
- 1 ounce chopped fresh dill
- 1½ ounces chopped fresh mint
- ¼ teaspoon kosher salt
- 6 ounces shredded iceberg lettuce
- 1 tomato (5 ounces), diced

To make the chicken: Combine the oil, lemon juice, oregano, salt, and pepper in a shallow dish; add the chicken. Refrigerate for 2–3 hours. Drain and discard the marinade.

Grill the chicken until a thermometer inserted in the thickest portion registers 160°F and the juices run clear. Refrigerate until chilled.

To make the sauce: Combine the yogurt, cucumbers, garlic, oil, vinegar, dill, mint, and salt. Process in a blender or food processor until smooth. Refrigerate until chilled.

To serve, julienne the chicken and arrange on a bed of lettuce. Place the tomato pieces on top. Serve with the sauce.

Serves 4

NUTRITION AT A GLANCE

Per serving: 281 calories, 30 g protein, 10 g carbohydrates, 14 g fat, 2 g saturated fats, 355 mg sodium, 67 mg cholesterol, 1 g fiber

South Beach Salad

Vinaigrette Dressing

- 3 tablespoons extra-virgin olive oil
- 3 tablespoons vegetable oil
- 3 tablespoons wine vinegar
- ½ teaspoon Dijon mustard
- ½ teaspoon salt
- ½ teaspoon freshly ground black pepper

Salad

- 1 can (14 ounces) hearts of palm, drained and sliced
- ½ cup chopped green bell pepper
- ½ cup chopped red bell pepper
- 1 can (14 ounces) artichoke hearts, drained and quartered
- 10 pimiento-stuffed olives, halved
- 1 head Boston lettuce
- 2 hard-cooked eggs, quartered
- 12 cherry tomatoes, halved

To make the vinaigrette dressing: Combine the olive oil, vegetable oil, vinegar, mustard, salt, and pepper in a screw-top jar. Cover tightly and shake vigorously to mix.

To make the salad: Combine the hearts of palm, peppers, artichoke hearts, and olives in a bowl. Add the vinaigrette dressing and mix well. Refrigerate for at least 1 hour.

To serve, place the salad on a bed of lettuce leaves and garnish with the egg and cherry tomatoes.

Serves 6

NUTRITION AT A GLANCE

Per serving: 226 calories, 7 g protein, 15 g carbohydrates, 17 g fat, 2 g saturated fats, 710 mg sodium, 71 mg cholesterol, 6 g fiber

Perfection Salad

1 envelope Knox unflavored gelatin

½ + 1¼ cups water

¼ cup Equal sweetener

¼ cup white vinegar

½ teaspoon salt

¾ cup finely shredded cabbage

1 cup diced celery

1 pimiento, chopped

In a saucepan, sprinkle the gelatin on ½ cup of the water to soften. Cook over low heat and stir until the gelatin is dissolved. Remove from the heat. Add the sugar substitute, the remaining water, the vinegar, and the salt. Chill to unbeaten egg-white consistency.

Fold in the cabbage, celery, and pimiento. Turn into a 3-cup mold or individual molds and chill until firm.

Serves 6

NUTRITION AT A GLANCE

Per serving: 44 calories, 2 g protein, 9 g carbohydrates, 0 g fat, 0 g saturated fats, 219 mg sodium, 0 mg cholesterol, 1 g fiber

From the Menu of . . .

MACALUSO'S

1747 Alton Road, Miami Beach

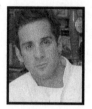

EXECUTIVE CHEF/OWNER: **MICHAEL D'ANDREA**

MACALUSO'S–THE ONLY RESTAURANT IN SOUTH FLORIDA
SERVING HOME–COOKED ITALIAN FOOD FROM
STATEN ISLAND, NEW YORK.

Macaluso's Salad

2–3 romaine lettuce hearts, cut into 1" pieces

1 red bell pepper, cut into 1" pieces

1 cucumber, thinly sliced

1 medium tomato, cut into eighths

¼ cup red onion, thinly sliced and cut into 1-inch pieces

¼ cup extra-virgin olive oil, first cold-pressed

¼ cup very fine red wine vinegar

3 teaspoons grated Romano cheese

Salt

Freshly ground black pepper

¼ cup canned chickpeas

Place the romaine hearts, bell pepper, cucumber, tomato, and onion in a salad bowl.

Combine the olive oil, red wine vinegar, cheese, salt, and pepper in a screw-top jar and shake well. Drizzle the dressing over the salad. Add the chickpeas and toss well.

Serves 2

NUTRITION AT A GLANCE
Per serving: 389 calories, 9 g protein, 25 g carbohydrates, 30 g fat, 5 g saturated fats, 153 mg sodium, 3 mg cholesterol, 9 g fiber

White Asparagus Salad

1 teaspoon chopped fresh tarragon

½ cup finely chopped, seeded tomatoes

⅓ cup extra-virgin olive oil

1 clove garlic, minced

2 tablespoons white wine vinegar

Lettuce leaves

1 jar (12 ounces) white asparagus spears, drained

In a small bowl, combine the tarragon, tomatoes, oil, garlic, and vinegar.

To serve, place the lettuce leaves on individual serving plates. Arrange 4–6 asparagus spears on the lettuce leaves. Spoon about 3 tablespoons of the vinaigrette over the asparagus on each plate.

Serves 4

NUTRITION AT A GLANCE

Per serving: 193 calories, 2 g protein,
5 g carbohydrates, 19 g fat, 3 g saturated fats,
247 mg sodium, 0 mg cholesterol, 2 g fiber

Zucchini Ribbons with Dill

4 medium zucchini (about 1½ pounds) sliced lengthwise into ribbons

2 tablespoons grated Parmesan cheese

2 tablespoons fresh dill, chopped

1 tablespoon extra-virgin olive oil

1 teaspoon red-pepper flakes

Bring a pot of water to a boil. Add the zucchini to the boiling water and cook for 30–60 seconds, or until tender-crisp. Drain.

Transfer the zucchini to a serving bowl. Add the Parmesan cheese, dill, oil, and red-pepper flakes. Gently toss until the zucchini is coated.

Serves 4

NUTRITION AT A GLANCE

Per serving: 68 calories, 3 g protein,
5 g carbohydrates, 5 g fat, 1 g saturated fats,
52 mg sodium, 2 mg cholesterol, 2 g fiber

Vegetable Medley

1   medium zucchini, cut into bite-size pieces

1   medium summer squash, cut into bite-size pieces

1   medium red bell pepper, cut into bite-size pieces

1   medium yellow bell pepper, cut into bite-size pieces

1   pound fresh asparagus, cut into bite-size pieces

1   red onion, cut into bite-size pieces

3   tablespoons olive oil

1   teaspoon salt

½   teaspoon fresh ground black pepper

Heat the oven to 450°F. In a large roasting pan, combine the zucchini, squash, red and yellow peppers, asparagus, and onion. Add the olive oil, salt, and black pepper. Toss to mix and coat. Spread in a single layer.

Roast for 30 minutes, stirring occasionally, until the vegetables are lightly browned and tender.

Serves 4

NUTRITION AT A GLANCE

Per serving: 169 calories, 5 g protein,
15 g carbohydrates, 11 g fat, 2 g saturated fats,
590 mg sodium, 0 mg cholesterol, 5 g fiber

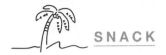 SNACK

Baba Ghannouj

- 1 medium eggplant, peeled
- 1 clove garlic, minced
- 1 tablespoon tahini (sesame paste)
- ⅛ teaspoon ground cumin

    Assorted raw vegetables

Preheat the broiler. Slice the eggplant crosswise into ½" slices. Place the slices on a baking sheet and broil 3" from the heat until soft and water beads on the surface. Cool and peel the slices. Puree in a blender or food processor along with the garlic, tahini, and cumin.

Chill and serve with vegetables.

Serves 1

NUTRITION AT A GLANCE

Per serving: 213 calories, 8 g protein,
32 g carbohydrates, 9 g fat, 1 g saturated fats,
20 mg sodium, 0 mg cholesterol, 12 g fiber

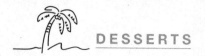

DESSERTS

Chocolate-Dipped Strawberries

2   squares (1 ounce each) semisweet or bittersweet chocolate,
    chopped

½   tablespoon whipping cream

    Dash almond extract

8   strawberries

Combine the chocolate and the whipping cream in a glass measuring cup
or bowl. Microwave at medium power for 1 minute or until the
chocolate melts, stirring after 30 seconds. Stir in the almond extract and
cool slightly.

Dip each strawberry into the melted chocolate, allowing the excess to
drip off. Place on a waxed paper–lined baking sheet. Refrigerate or
freeze for approximately 15 minutes until the chocolate is set.

Serves 2

NUTRITION AT A GLANCE

Per serving: 175 calories, 3 g protein,
24 g carbohydrates, 9 g fat, 6 g saturated fats,
1 mg sodium, 5 mg cholesterol, 4 g fiber

Strawberries with Vanilla Yogurt

4 ounces non-fat, sugar-free vanilla yogurt

½ cup chopped strawberries

Spoon the yogurt into a parfait glass, then add the strawberries.
Serve immediately.

Serves 1

NUTRITION AT A GLANCE

Per serving: 85 calories, 4 g protein,
16 g carbohydrates, 0 g fat, 0 g saturated fats,
66 mg sodium, 3 mg cholesterol, 2 g fiber

Pistachio Bark

12 squares semisweet chocolate

1 cup pistachio nuts, shelled and toasted

Microwave the chocolate in a microwaveable bowl on high for 2 minutes,
stirring after 1 minute. Stir until completely melted. Stir the nuts into the
chocolate.

Spoon the chocolate and nut mixture onto a waxed paper–lined
baking sheet. Refrigerate for 1 hour until firm. Break into bite-size
pieces.

Makes approximately 40 individual servings

NUTRITION AT A GLANCE

Per ounce: 150 calories, 3 g protein,
16 g carbohydrates, 10 g fat, 4 g saturated fats,
0 mg sodium, 0 mg cholesterol, 2 g fiber

Chocolate Cups

1 package (3½ ounces) sugar-free vanilla pudding mix

1¼ cups fat-free milk

¾ cup lite frozen whipped topping, thawed

8 Astor Chocolate Liqueur Cups (available at liquor stores)

Cocoa powder

Prepare the pudding using the milk. With a rubber spatula, fold in the whipped topping. Spoon the cream filling into the chocolate cups. Sprinkle with cocoa powder.

Serves 8

NUTRITION AT A GLANCE

Per serving: 99 calories, 2 g protein,
17 g carbohydrates, 3 g fat, 1 g saturated fats,
206 mg sodium, 5 mg cholesterol, 0 g fiber

PHASE
THREE
Meal Plan

By now you should be at your ideal weight. If you've stuck with the diet, your blood chemistry should also be improved. This is the part of the plan that's meant to help you maintain the benefits you've earned by following phases 1 and 2. This is how you'll eat for the rest of your life. Phase 3 is the most liberal stage of the diet—by now it is simply one important aspect of a healthy lifestyle rather than a weight-loss program. At this point you should be knowledgeable enough about how the South Beach Diet works and how it interacts with your own body to enjoy all the flexibility of the plan. That's why there's no food list for Phase Three. In other words, if you want it, and it doesn't undo all your sacrifices, you should go ahead and enjoy. There will always be times when you overindulge a little, even after years on the diet. Those are the times when you'll switch back to Phase 1 for a week or two. You'll get back to where you were, and then you'll return to Phase 3. Don't even think of it as backsliding—we designed the diet to allow normal human beings to eat the way they want. If for you, that means having a few too many desserts once in a while, great. Enjoy it.

Day 1

Breakfast

½ grapefruit

2 Vegetable Quiche Cups to Go (page 134)

Oatmeal (½ cup old-fashioned oatmeal mixed with1 cup nonfat milk, cooked on low heat, and sprinkled with cinnamon and 1 Tbsp chopped walnuts)

Decaffeinated coffee or decaffeinated tea with nonfat milk and sugar substitute

Lunch

Roast Beef Wrap (page 265)

Fresh apple

Dinner

Moroccan Grilled Chicken (page 266)

Steamed asparagus

Couscous

Mediterranean Salad (page 286)

Olive oil and vinegar to taste or 2 Tbsp low-sugar prepared dressing

Dessert

Strawberries with Vanilla Yogurt (page 241)

Day 2

Breakfast

Fresh orange, sliced

¼–½ cup liquid egg substitute

2 slices Canadian bacon

1 slice whole grain bread

Decaffeinated coffee or decaffeinated tea with nonfat milk and sugar substitute

Lunch

South Beach Chopped Salad with Tuna (page 140)

Sugar-free flavored gelatin dessert

Dinner

Stir-Fry Chicken and Vegetables (page 215)

Asian Style Cabbage Salad (page 177)

Dessert

Lemon Zest Ricotta Crème (page 180)

Day 3

Breakfast

½ grapefruit

Egg white omelet with salsa

1 slice multigrain bread

Decaffeinated coffee or decaffeinated tea with nonfat milk and sugar substitute

Lunch

Open-faced ham and Swiss cheese sandwich on rye

1 fresh apple

Dinner

Broiled sirloin steak

Creamed Spinach (page 280)

Surprise South Beach Mashed "Potatoes" (page 171)

Fresh Mozzarella–Tomato Salad (page 281)

Dessert

Chocolate-Dipped Apricots (page 294)

Day 4

Breakfast

½ grapefruit

Oatmeal (½ cup old-fashioned oatmeal mixed with1 cup nonfat milk, cooked on low heat, and sprinkled with cinnamon and 1 Tbsp chopped walnuts)

1 poached egg

1 slice multigrain bread

1 tablespoon low-sugar fruit spread

Decaffeinated coffee or decaffeinated tea with nonfat milk and sugar substitute

Lunch

Tomato stuffed with chicken salad

Fresh melon wedge

4 oz non-fat, sugar-free yogurt

Dinner

Snapper Provençal (page 274)

Steamed snow peas

Rice pilaf

Tossed salad (mixed greens, cucumbers, green peppers, cherry tomatoes)

Olive oil and vinegar to taste or 2 Tbsp low-sugar prepared dressing

Dessert

Chocolate-Stuffed Steamed Pears (page 293)

Day 5

Breakfast

½ grapefruit

Western Egg White Omelet (page 133)

½ whole wheat English muffin

Decaffeinated coffee or decaffeinated tea with nonfat milk and sugar substitute

Lunch

Greek Salad (page 137)

4 oz non-fat, sugar-free raspberry yogurt

Dinner

Beef, Pepper, and Mushroom Kabobs (page 273)

Brown rice

Avocado and tomato salad

Olive oil and vinegar to taste

Dessert

Almond Ricotta Crème (page 181)

Day 6

Breakfast

Fresh blueberries

Cinnamon Surprise (page 260)

Decaffeinated coffee or decaffeinated tea with nonfat milk and sugar substitute

Lunch

Chicken Caesar Salad (no croutons)

2 Tbsp prepared Caesar dressing

Dinner

Savory Shrimp over Wild Rice (page 277)

Arugula salad

2 Tbsp Balsamic Vinaigrette (page 148) or low-sugar prepared dressing

Dessert

Swiss Knight Fondue au Chocolate with fresh strawberries

Day 7

Breakfast

Fresh orange, sliced

Tomato and Herb Frittata (page 259)

1 slice multigrain toast

1 Tbsp low-sugar fruit spread

Decaffeinated coffee or decaffeinated tea with nonfat milk and sugar substitute

Lunch

Tuna, Cucumber, and Red Pepper Salad with Lemony Dill Dressing (page 264)

Sugar-free flavored gelatin dessert

Dinner

Apricot-Glazed Cornish Hens (page 271)

Couscous

Bibb lettuce salad

Olive oil and balsamic vinegar to taste or 2 Tbsp prepared low-sugar dressing

Dessert

Chocolate Sponge Cake (page 292)

Day 8

Breakfast

6 oz vegetable juice cocktail

¼–½ cup liquid egg substitute

1 slice Canadian bacon

½ whole wheat English muffin

1 tsp low-sugar fruit spread

Decaffeinated coffee or decaffeinated tea with nonfat milk and sugar substitute

Lunch

Grilled chicken salad

2 Tbsp Balsamic Vinaigrette (page 148) or low-sugar prepared dressing

Dinner

Grilled Rosemary Steak (page 272)

Fresh steamed green beans

Baked Tomatoes with Basil and Parmesan (page 230)

Arugula and Watercress Salad (page 282)

2 Tbsp Balsamic Vinaigrette (page 148) or low-sugar prepared dressing

Dessert

Fresh strawberries and blueberries in Chocolate Cups (page 242)

Day 9

Breakfast

Fresh orange, sliced

2 Vegetable Quiche Cups to Go (page 134)

1 slice multigrain toast

Decaffeinated coffee or decaffeinated tea with nonfat milk and sugar substitute

Lunch

Couscous Salad with Spicy Yogurt Dressing (page 262)

Fresh nectarine

Dinner

Lemony Fish in Foil (page 275)

Zucchini with dill

Sliced tomato

Sliced cantaloupe

Dessert

Strawberries in Balsamic Vinegar (page 288)

Day 10

Breakfast

½ grapefruit

Oatmeal Pancake (page 201)

Decaffeinated coffee or decaffeinated tea with nonfat milk and sugar substitute

Lunch

Open-faced roast beef sandwich (3 oz lean roast beef, lettuce, tomato, onion, mustard, 1 slice whole grain bread)

Small Granny Smith apple

Dinner

Baked chicken breast

Italian-Style Spaghetti Squash (page 229)

Tossed salad (mixed greens, cucumbers, green peppers, cherry tomatoes)

Prepared low-sugar Italian dressing

Dessert

Sliced nectarines and fresh blueberries with 4 oz non-fat, sugar-free vanilla yogurt

Day 11

Breakfast

Berry smoothie (8 oz non-fat, sugar-free fruit-flavored yogurt, ½ cup berries, ½ cup crushed ice; blend until smooth)

Decaffeinated coffee or decaffeinated tea with nonfat milk and sugar substitute

Lunch

Endive and Pecan Salad (page 261)

Turkey-tomato pita (3 oz sliced turkey, 3 tomato slices, ½ cup shredded lettuce, 1 tsp Dijon mustard in a whole wheat pita)

4 oz non-fat, sugar-free lemon yogurt

Dinner

Marinated London Broil (page 158)

Grilled asparagus and peppers

Herb-roasted new potatoes

Tossed salad (mixed greens, cucumbers, green peppers, cherry tomatoes)

Olive oil and vinegar to taste or 2 Tbsp low-sugar prepared dressing

Dessert

Individual Lime Cheesecakes (page 291)

Day 12

Breakfast

½ fresh grapefruit

Tex-Mex eggs (2 eggs scrambled with shredded Monterey Jack cheese and salsa)

1 slice whole grain toast

Decaffeinated coffee or decaffeinated tea with nonfat milk and sugar substitute

Lunch

Roast Beef Wrap (London broil left over from Day 11) (page 265)

Fresh nectarine

Dinner

Grilled salmon with tomato salsa

Grilled asparagus

Tossed salad (mixed greens, cucumbers, green peppers, cherry tomatoes)

Olive oil and vinegar to taste or 2 Tbsp low-sugar prepared dressing

Dessert

Chocolate-Dipped Apricots (page 294)

Day 13

Breakfast

½ grapefruit

Light Spinach Frittata with Tomato Salsa (page 130)

Decaffeinated coffee or decaffeinated tea with nonfat milk and sugar substitute

Lunch

Cottage cheese and chopped vegetables in red pepper cup

Sliced cantaloupe with blueberries

Dinner

Tandoori Cornish Hens (page 270)

Endive and Pecan Salad (page 261)

Couscous

Hummus (page 178) with pita chips and fresh vegetables

(May use store-bought hummus)

Dessert

Pear poached in dry red wine

Day 14

Breakfast

South Beach Blintz (1 egg beaten with ⅓ cup crumbled farmer cheese and Splenda to taste, fried in nonstick omelet pan with cooking spray)

Decaffeinated coffee or decaffeinated tea with nonfat milk and sugar substitute

Lunch

Chef's salad (at least 1 oz each ham, turkey, and low-fat Swiss cheese on mixed greens)

Olive oil and vinegar to taste or 2 Tbsp low-sugar prepared dressing

1 slice whole grain bread

Dinner

Lime-Baked Fish (page 276)

Broiled Tomatoes (page 173)

Steamed Brussels sprouts

Artichoke salad (chilled cooked artichoke hearts with halved cherry tomatoes and chopped scallions)

2 Tbsp Balsamic Vinaigrette (page 148) or low-sugar prepared dressing

Dessert

Chocolate-Dipped Strawberries (page 240)

PHASE THREE
Recipes

Once you've reached your goal you'll switch to these recipes, which now include foods such as multigrain bread, tortillas, and brown rice. At this point you'll know which carbs you can eat without gaining weight, so you'll have already integrated them into your diet. You'll notice that by this phase we've put an end to the two daytime snacks—by now you shouldn't really need them to keep you satisfied between meals. But this is also the phase that includes Chocolate Sponge Cake, which is a fair trade.

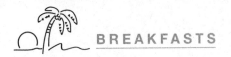

BREAKFASTS

Tomato and Herb Frittata

½ cup chopped plum tomatoes

¼ cup chopped scallions

3 basil leaves, chopped

1 tablespoon I Can't Believe It's Not Butter! Spray

1 cup liquid egg substitute

Coat an ovenproof 10" skillet with cooking spray and place over medium heat until hot. Sauté the tomatoes, scallions, and basil in the butter until tender. Reduce the heat to low. Pour the egg substitute evenly into the skillet over the mixture. Cover and cook for 5–7 minutes or until cooked on the bottom and almost set on the top.

Transfer the skillet to a broiler and broil until the top is set, 2–3 minutes. Slide onto a serving platter and cut into wedges to serve.

Serves 2

NUTRITION AT A GLANCE

Per serving: 169 calories, 16 g protein, 5 g carbohydrates, 9 g fat, 2 g saturated fats, 278 mg sodium, 1 mg cholesterol, 1 g fiber

Cinnamon Surprise

¼ cup low-fat cottage cheese

1 slice multigrain bread

   Dash cinnamon

Spread the cottage cheese onto the slice of bread. Sprinkle with the cinnamon and broil until bubbly, 2–3 minutes.

Serves 1

NUTRITION AT A GLANCE

Per serving: 87 calories, 9 g protein,
12 g carbohydrates, 1 g fat, 0 g saturated fats,
347 mg sodium, 5 mg cholesterol, 3 g fiber

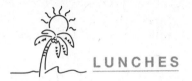

LUNCHES

Endive and Pecan Salad

3 cups loosely packed Boston lettuce

1 onion, sliced

3 cups loosely packed curly endive

¼ teaspoon freshly ground black pepper

¾ cup coarsely chopped pecans, toasted

¼ cup red wine vinegar

¼ teaspoon salt

Combine the lettuce, onion, endive, and pepper in a large bowl. Set aside.
   Add the pecans, vinegar, and salt to a skillet and cook over low heat
until thoroughly heated. Pour over the lettuce and toss gently.

Serves 6

NUTRITION AT A GLANCE

Per serving: 118 calories, 2 g protein,
7 g carbohydrates, 10 g fat, 1 g saturated fats,
101 mg sodium, 0 mg cholesterol, 3 g fiber

Couscous Salad with Spicy Yogurt Dressing

Couscous

- 1 tablespoon extra-virgin olive oil
- 1 small onion, finely chopped
- 1 small rib celery, finely chopped
- 1 cup couscous
- 1½ cups water

Spicy Yogurt Dressing

- 3 tablespoons fresh lemon juice
- 3 tablespoons fat-free plain yogurt
- 1 tablespoon extra-virgin olive oil
- 2 teaspoons minced fresh gingerroot
- 1 clove garlic, crushed
- 1 teaspoon ground cumin
- 1 teaspoon ground coriander
- Pinch freshly ground black pepper

Salad

- ½ cup dried currants or raisins
- ½ cup canned chickpeas, rinsed and drained
- ½ cup chopped red bell pepper
- ½ cup chopped green bell pepper
- ½ cup chopped fresh cilantro or parsley
- ½ cup sliced medium scallions
- 1 lemon, cut into wedges (optional)

To make the couscous: Heat the oil in a 2-quart saucepan over medium heat. Add the onion and celery and cook for 2–3 minutes, stirring occasionally, until the vegetables are softened. Stir in the couscous, coating with oil. Cook and stir for 1 minute until lightly toasted. Add the water and bring to a boil, stirring gently. Remove from the heat. Let stand, covered, for 30 minutes until cool and the liquid is absorbed, uncovering occasionally to fluff with a fork.

To make the spicy yogurt dressing: In a large bowl, mix together the lemon juice, yogurt, oil, gingerroot, garlic, cumin, coriander, and pepper. Whisk before serving.

To make the salad: Transfer the couscous to a large serving bowl. Spoon the currants, chickpeas, bell peppers, cilantro or parsley, and scallions into separate mounds around the couscous. Add the dressing. Toss all the ingredients together at the table. Garnish with the lemon wedges, if using.

Serves 4

NUTRITION AT A GLANCE

Per serving: 393 calories, 12 g protein, 69 g carbohydrates, 9 g fat, 1 g saturated fats, 31 mg sodium, 1 mg cholesterol, 8 g fiber

Tuna, Cucumber, and Red Pepper Salad with Lemony Dill Dressing

Lemony Dill Dressing

- ¼ cup extra virgin olive oil
- 3 tablespoons fresh lemon juice
- 1–2 tablespoons chopped fresh dill
- ½ teaspoon salt
- ½ teaspoon coarsely ground black pepper

Salad

- 2 medium cucumbers, chopped
- 1 red bell pepper, chopped
- 2 cans (6.5 ounces each) solid white tuna, drained and flaked

  Romaine lettuce
- 1 small lemon, peeled, seeded, and sliced

To make the lemony dill dressing: Whisk the olive oil, lemon juice, dill, salt, and black pepper together in a small bowl.

To make the salad: Combine the cucumbers, bell pepper, and tuna in a large bowl. Set aside. Arrange the lettuce on 4 plates. Spoon the tuna mixture into the center of each plate. Arrange the lemon around the plates. Drizzle with the dressing.

Serves 4

NUTRITION AT A GLANCE

Per serving: 282 calories, 24 g protein, 9 g carbohydrates, 17 g fat, 3 g saturated fats, 640 mg sodium, 39 mg cholesterol, 2 g fiber

Roast Beef Wrap

¼ cup reduced-fat cream cheese

4 9"–10" flour tortillas

½ red onion, sliced

4 spinach leaves, washed

8 ounces sliced roast beef

For each wrap, spread a small amount of the cream cheese over the surface of a tortilla. Layer the onion, spinach, and roast beef on top. Fold opposite sides of the tortilla toward the center about 1½" and roll up from the bottom.

Serves 4

NUTRITION AT A GLANCE

Per serving: 300 calories, 13 g protein, 42 g carbohydrates, 9 g fat, 3 g saturated fats, 659 mg sodium, 21 mg cholesterol, 3 g fiber

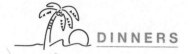 DINNERS

Moroccan Grilled Chicken

¼ cup extra-virgin olive oil

1 teaspoon dried oregano

½ teaspoon ground allspice

½ teaspoon ground cumin

½ teaspoon ground cloves

3 cloves garlic, minced

4 boneless, skinless chicken breast halves

1 box (5.8 ounces) Near East couscous

   Red Pimiento Sauce (page 267)

Combine the oil, oregano, allspice, cumin, cloves, and garlic in a large
bowl. Add the chicken breasts and cover with the olive oil mixture. Cook
on a preheated grill over medium heat for about 30 minutes or until the
juices run clear when the chicken is pierced. Remove from the grill and
keep warm.

     Meanwhile, prepare the couscous according to package directions.
When the couscous is ready, divide it among 4 plates. Thinly slice
each chicken breast and fan over the couscous on each plate. Drizzle
2 tablespoons of the sauce over each chicken breast.

Serves 4

NUTRITION AT A GLANCE

> **Per serving:** 429 calories, 32 g protein,
> 37 g carbohydrates, 16 g fat, 2 g saturated fats,
> 89 mg sodium, 66 mg cholesterol, 4 g fiber

Red Pimiento Sauce

½ cup canned pimientos, drained

2 tablespoons lemon juice

Combine the pimientos and lemon juice in a food processor. Process
for 30–45 seconds or until the sauce is smooth. Transfer to a covered
container. Serve at room temperature.

Makes 8 tablespoons

NUTRITION AT A GLANCE

Per serving: 10 calories, 0 g protein,
2 g carbohydrates, 0 g fat, 0 g saturated fats,
4 mg sodium, 0 mg cholesterol, 0 g fiber

RUMI SUPPER CLUB

330 Lincoln Road, Miami Beach

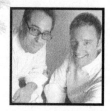

EXECUTIVE CHEFS: **SCOTT FREDEL**
and **J. D. HARRIS**

Roast Chicken with Sweet Garlic, Melted Onions, and Sour Orange

3	pounds chicken
½	cup whole garlic cloves, peeled
1	cup + 3 tablespoons olive oil
1	bunch flat-leaf parsley
	Zest of 1 orange
	Zest of 1 lime
1	pound yuca, peeled
2	Spanish onions, thinly sliced
16	ounces sour orange juice
1	cup rich chicken stock

Cut the chicken in half and debone. Place the garlic in ¼ cup of the oil and sauté until tender. When the garlic is cool, puree half of it with the parsley, orange zest, lime zest, and the remaining ¾ cup of oil. Rub the garlic mixture onto the chicken and marinate for 1 day in the refrigerator.

Cook the yuca in salted water until tender, and drain. Slowly cook the onions with a little water until soft. Reserve.

Simmer the sour orange juice over low heat until syrupy. Add the chicken stock and cook until lightly thickened. Reserve.

Bake the chicken at 350°F for 45 minutes, until cooked through and the juices run clear when pierced with a fork. Sauté the yuca in the remaining 3 tablespoons olive oil until crispy. Add the onions and the reserved garlic confit.

Drain the yuca mixture well and place on a plate with the chicken. Cover with the orange mixture.

Yuca is a root vegetable readily available in South Florida owing mainly to our South American and Caribbean influences. Use the drained oil sparingly for flavoring while maintaining or losing weight. Remember, sauté, don't fry!

Sour orange juice comes from Caribbean sour oranges known as naranjas. If unavailable, mix ½ cup lemon juice with 1½ cups orange juice.

Serves 6

NUTRITION AT A GLANCE
Per serving: 630 calories, 25 g protein, 50 g carbohydrates, 37 g fat, 8 g saturated fats, 240 mg sodium, 85 mg cholesterol, 4 g fiber

Tandoori Cornish Hens

3 Cornish hens, approximately 1 pound each
1½ teaspoons chili powder
½ teaspoon salt (optional)
  Pinch freshly ground black pepper
3 tablespoons fresh lime juice
1 cup fat-free plain yogurt
3 cloves garlic, chopped
1 inch fresh ginger, coarsely chopped
1 small onion, coarsely chopped
1 teaspoon cumin seeds
½ teaspoon ground turmeric
1 lime, cut into wedges (optional)
  Fresh cilantro or parsley sprigs (optional)

Thaw the hens if frozen. Rinse, remove the giblets and necks, and pat dry. Make several slits in the skin, then split each hen in half along the breastbone.

Mix together 1 teaspoon of the chili powder, salt, pepper, and lime juice. Rub the mixture all over the poultry and set aside for about 15 minutes.

In a blender, puree the yogurt, garlic, ginger, onion, cumin, turmeric, and the remaining ½ teaspoon of chili powder. Place the poultry pieces in a bowl and add the yogurt mixture. Mix well to coat all the pieces. Cover and refrigerate for at least 8 hours, turning occasionally.

Preheat the oven to 400°F. Place the hens, skin side up, on a rack in a roasting pan. Spoon the yogurt mixture over them from time to time until thoroughly cooked, 45–60 minutes or until the hens are very tender. Test for doneness by pricking the skin of the thigh; the juice should run clear. Serve hot.

Remove the skin before eating, and garnish with lime and cilantro or parsley, if using.

Serves 6

NUTRITION AT A GLANCE

Per serving: 150 calories, 22 g protein,
8 g carbohydrates, 4 g fat, 1 g saturated fats,
100 mg sodium, 90 mg cholesterol, 1 g fiber

Apricot-Glazed Cornish Hens

1   cup Smuckers Light Sugar-Free Apricot Preserves

⅓   cup fresh orange juice

¼   cup I Can't Believe It's Not Butter! Spray

4   Cornish hens, thawed

     Pinch salt

     Pinch freshly ground black pepper

Combine the preserves, orange juice, and butter to make the glaze. Rinse the hens and pat dry. Rub the cavities with salt and pepper. Place the hens, breast sides up, on a rack in a roasting pan, ensuring that they do not touch. Pour on the glaze. Roast for 1 hour at 350°F, basting every 10 minutes or until the hens are very tender. Test for doneness by pricking the skin of the thigh; the juice should run clear.

Remove the hens from the oven and let stand for 10 minutes before serving.

Serves 4

NUTRITION AT A GLANCE

Per serving: 449 calories, 22 g protein,
26 g carbohydrates, 28 g fat, 7 g saturated fats,
171 mg sodium, 126 mg cholesterol, 1 g fiber

Grilled Rosemary Steak

4 boneless beef loins or New York strip steaks

2 tablespoons fresh rosemary leaves, minced

2 cloves garlic, minced

1 tablespoon extra-virgin olive oil

1 teaspoon grated lemon peel

1 teaspoon coarsely ground black pepper

   Fresh rosemary sprigs (optional)

Score the steaks in a diamond pattern on both sides. Mix the fresh rosemary, garlic, oil, lemon peel, and black pepper in a small bowl. Rub the mixture onto the surface of the steaks. Cover and refrigerate for 1 hour.

Grill the steaks until a thermometer inserted in the center registers 145°F (for medium-rare). Cut the steaks diagonally into ½" thick slices. Garnish with the rosemary sprigs, if using.

Serves 4

NUTRITION AT A GLANCE

Per serving: 247 calories, 21 g protein,
1 g carbohydrates, 17 g fat, 6 g saturated fats,
50 mg sodium, 60 mg cholesterol, 0 g fiber

Beef, Pepper, and Mushroom Kabobs

1 tablespoon fresh lemon juice

1 tablespoon extra-virgin olive oil

1 tablespoon water

2 teaspoons Dijon mustard

½ teaspoon chopped fresh oregano

¼ teaspoon freshly ground black pepper

1 pound boneless top sirloin steak, cut into 1" squares

1 large red bell pepper, cut into 1" pieces

12 large mushrooms

2 cups cooked brown rice

¼ cup pine nuts, toasted

In a large bowl, whisk together the lemon juice, oil, water, mustard, oregano, and black pepper. Add the steak, bell pepper, and mushrooms, tossing to coat. Alternately thread the steak, bell pepper, and mushrooms on each of 4 metal skewers. Set aside.

Prepare the rice according to package directions. Keep warm. Meanwhile, place the kabobs on a grill over medium coals. Grill uncovered, turning occasionally for 8–11 minutes or until a meat thermometer measures 145°F (for medium-rare).

Mix the toasted pine nuts into the rice. Serve the kabobs over the rice mixture, allowing ½ cup rice per serving.

Serves 4

NUTRITION AT A GLANCE

Per serving: 493 calories, 33 g protein, 50 g carbohydrates, 18 g fat, 5 g saturated fats, 125 mg sodium, 75 mg cholesterol, 4 g fiber

Snapper Provençal

¼ cup extra-virgin olive oil

1½ pounds fresh red snapper fillets

⅓ cup kalamata olives

2½ tablespoons capers

1 cup canned tomatoes

3 tablespoons chopped shallots

½ tablespoon fresh rosemary leaves

½ tablespoon minced garlic

⅓ cup white wine

Preheat the oven to 450°F. Preheat a large sauté pan on high heat for
2–3 minutes. Pour the oil into the pan, swirling to coat. Add the snapper
to the pan and lower the heat to medium-high. Sauté the snapper for
6–10 minutes, turning once halfway through the cooking time. Remove
the snapper from the pan when it flakes easily. Gently slide the fillets onto
a baking sheet. Place in the oven to keep warm. Combine the olives,
capers, tomatoes, and shallots in the pan. Stir in the rosemary and garlic,
add the wine, and sauté for 5 minutes. Remove the fillets from the oven,
place on a serving platter and pour the vegetable mixture over the top.

Serves 4

NUTRITION AT A GLANCE

Per serving: 362 calories, 36 g protein,
6 g carbohydrates, 19 g fat, 3 g saturated fats,
543 mg sodium, 63 mg cholesterol, 1 g fiber

Lemony Fish in Foil

4 large fish fillets

¼ cup diced carrots

¼ cup diced celery

¼ cup chopped green onion

2 tablespoons chopped fresh parsley

2 lemons, thinly sliced

Heat the oven to 350°F. Cut four 2-foot lengths of foil and fold each in half to make a 1-foot square. Place 1 fish fillet slightly below the middle of each square of foil. Sprinkle ¼ of the carrots, celery, green onion, and parsley on each fillet. Top with lemon slices.

Fold the foil over the fish and crimp the edges together slightly. Place the foil-wrapped fillets on a baking sheet and bake for 15–20 minutes or until the fish flakes easily.

Serves 2

NUTRITION AT A GLANCE

Per serving: 119 calories, 22 g protein,
5 g carbohydrates, 1 g fat, 0 g saturated fats,
97 mg sodium, 65 mg cholesterol, 1 g fiber

Lime-Baked Fish

½ pound fresh fish fillets

¼ cup fresh lime juice

1 teaspoon tarragon leaves

¼ cup chopped green onion tops

Preheat the oven to 325°F. Arrange the fish fillets in a baking dish. Sprinkle with the lime juice, tarragon, and onion tops. Bake, covered, at 325°F for 15–20 minutes or until the fish flakes easily.

Serves 2

NUTRITION AT A GLANCE

Per serving: 114 calories, 22 g protein,
4 g carbohydrates, 1 g fat, 0 g saturated fats,
80 mg sodium, 65 mg cholesterol, 1 g fiber

Savory Shrimp over Wild Rice

1   package (6 ounces) wild rice

1   pound shrimp, peeled and deveined

2   teaspoons paprika

½   teaspoon white pepper

½   teaspoon salt

½   clove garlic, minced

1   tablespoon extra-virgin olive oil

1   cup cherry tomatoes, halved

    Chopped fresh parsley (optional)

Prepare the wild rice according to the package directions.

In a large bowl, combine the shrimp, paprika, pepper, salt, and garlic. Mix well and set aside.

Heat the oil in a skillet until hot. Add the shrimp and cook on medium heat for 30 seconds. Stir in the tomatoes and cook for an additional 45 seconds or until the shrimp are opaque, stirring constantly. Remove from the heat and serve over ¼ cup of the wild rice. Garnish with parsley (if using).

Serves 4

NUTRITION AT A GLANCE

Per serving: 368 calories, 32 g protein,
46 g carbohydrates, 6 g fat, 1 g saturated fats,
467 mg sodium, 172 mg cholesterol, 4 g fiber

From the Menu of . . .

CHINA GRILL

404 Washington Avenue, Miami Beach

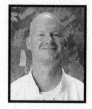

CHEF: CHRISTIAN PLOTCZYK

Asian Pear Salad

4 Asian pears, peeled, cored, and chopped

1 shallot, minced

2½ teaspoons diced fresh ginger

2 cups water

1 vanilla bean stick, scored in half

3 tablespoons sherry vinegar

2 tablespoons mirin (sweet sake)

¼ cup soybean oil

Salt

Black pepper

½ pound baby greens

1 carrot, shredded (optional)

In a 1-quart saucepan, cook the pears with the shallot, ginger, and water over medium heat until soft. Strain and set aside to cool. Once at room temperature, puree and strain through a sieve.

Remove the seeds from the vanilla bean and mix them into the puree. Discard the pods. Add the sherry vinegar and mirin and process in a blender or food processor. Slowly add the oil to emulsify. Season with the salt and pepper. Dice the remaining pear for garnish.

To serve, toss the baby greens well with the pear mixture. Divide among 4 serving plates and garnish with the shredded carrot (if using) and the diced pear.

This salad is served at China Grill accompanying their famous BBQ Lamb Ribs. Its delicious combination of ingredients makes it an innovative salad in tune with the South Beach Diet.

Serves 4

NUTRITION AT A GLANCE
Per serving: 200 calories, 2 g protein, 17 g carbohydrates, 14 g fat, 2 g saturated fats, 20 mg sodium, 0 mg cholesterol, 5 g fiber

Creamed Spinach

2 packages (10 ounces each) frozen spinach, thawed

2 small shallots, minced

1 clove garlic, minced

⅓ cup fat-free sour cream

½ teaspoon salt

¼ teaspoon coarsely ground black pepper

In a skillet, heat the spinach over medium-high heat for about 5 minutes or until the liquid evaporates. Add the shallots and garlic. Cook until tender. Reduce the heat to low. Add the sour cream, salt, and pepper, stirring until the sour cream melts. Do not simmer.

Serves 6

NUTRITION AT A GLANCE

Per serving: 35 calories, 3 g protein,
6 g carbohydrates, 0 g fat, 0 g saturated fats,
282 mg sodium, 0 mg cholesterol, 3 g fiber

Fresh Mozzarella-Tomato Salad

2 medium ripe tomatoes, sliced

4 ounces fresh mozzarella cheese, sliced

¼ cup fresh basil leaves

1 basil rosette

2 tablespoons extra-virgin olive oil

2 tablespoons balsamic vinegar

1 teaspoon cracked black pepper

Arrange the tomato, mozzarella, and basil in a rotating pattern on a large serving plate. Combine the oil and vinegar and drizzle over the salad. Sprinkle with the pepper.

Serves 4

NUTRITION AT A GLANCE

Per serving: 163 calories, 6 g protein, 5 g carbohydrates, 13 g fat, 5 g saturated fats, 114 mg sodium, 22 mg cholesterol, 1 g fiber

Arugula and Watercress Salad

Strawberry Preserves

5 ounces strawberries, stemmed and sliced

1 tablespoon balsamic vinegar

1½ tablespoons water

½ tablespoon cracked black pepper

Vinaigrette

1¼ tablespoons fresh lemon juice

1¼ tablespoons white wine vinegar

½ cup extra-virgin olive oil

1¼ tablespoons cracked black pepper

Salad

4 ounces arugula leaves

4 ounces watercress leaves

16 strawberries, stemmed and halved

Pinch freshly ground black pepper

To make the strawberry preserves: In a saucepan over medium heat, mix the strawberries, vinegar, water, and black pepper. Bring it to a boil and continue cooking at a low boil for 25 minutes, until slightly thickened, stirring occasionally. When cool, pour into a bowl, cover, and refrigerate.

To make the vinaigrette: In a medium bowl, mix together the lemon juice and vinegar. Whisk in the oil and pepper to blend thoroughly; cover and reserve. Whisk before serving.

To serve: In a large bowl, combine the arugula and watercress with the vinaigrette, reserving 4 tablespoons. Divide the mixture among 4 plates. Dip the cut sides of 4 strawberry halves in the pepper. Arrange them around the greens with 4 more strawberry halves. Dot each plate with 1 tablespoon of the reserved vinaigrette and 2 tablespoons of the preserves.

Serves 4

NUTRITION AT A GLANCE

Per serving: 308 calories, 2 g protein,
13 g carbohydrates, 28 g fat, 4 g saturated fats,
22 mg sodium, 0 mg cholesterol, 4 g fiber

From the Menu of . . .

MACALUSO'S

1747 Alton Road, Miami Beach

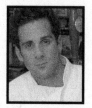

EXECUTIVE CHEF/OWNER: MICHAEL D'ANDREA

Macaluso's-Style Grilled Veal with Broccoli Rabe

Grilled Veal

- 1 teaspoon fresh chopped basil
- 2 cloves finely chopped garlic
- ¼ teaspoon paprika
- Salt
- Freshly ground black pepper
- 3 tablespoons finest extra-virgin olive oil, first cold-pressed
- 2 veal fillets (4 to 6 ounces each), thinly pounded

Broccoli Rabe

3 cups cleaned broccoli rabe (a healthy vegetable in the turnip family)

¼ cup extra-virgin olive oil, first cold pressed

¼ teaspoon freshly ground black pepper

¼ teaspoon salt

4 whole cloves garlic (peeled)

Pinch crushed red pepper

To make the grilled veal: Mix the basil, garlic, paprika, salt, and pepper with the olive oil. Place the veal in the mixture and hand stir. Place the veal on a grill and pour the remaining marinade on top. Grill over medium-high heat until done (approximately 3 minutes per side).

To make the broccoli rabe: Rinse the broccoli rabe in cold water and drain completely. Pour the oil, pepper, salt, garlic, and red pepper into a stock pot. Warm the oil over medium heat. Place the broccoli rabe in the pot, cover and cook for 4–7 minutes or until tender.

Place the cooked broccoli rabe on a plate and serve with the grilled veal on top.

Serves 2

NUTRITION AT A GLANCE
Per serving: 357 calories, 25 g protein, 9 g carbohydrates, 25 g fat, 4 g saturated fats, 380 mg sodium, 100 mg cholesterol, 0 g fiber

Mediterranean Salad

1 package prewashed romaine lettuce, torn into bite-size pieces

½ cup black olives, sliced

¼ cup feta cheese, crumbled

½ cup Balsamic Vinaigrette (page 148) or low-sugar prepared dressing

Combine the lettuce and the black olives in a large bowl. Toss well.
Divide the lettuce mixture onto 4 plates, sprinkle with the cheese, and
drizzle with the vinaigrette.

Serves 4

NUTRITION AT A GLANCE

Per serving: 101 calories, 2 g protein,
11 g carbohydrates, 5 g fat, 1 g saturated fats,
716 mg sodium, 8 mg cholesterol, 1 g fiber

Herbed Roasted Potatoes

1½ pounds small red potatoes

2 tablespoons extra-virgin olive oil

¾ teaspoon dried rosemary, crumbled

¾ teaspoon mustard powder

½ teaspoon dried sage

½ teaspoon dried thyme

¼ teaspoon pepper

Preheat the oven to 450°F or prepare the grill for direct heat. With a vegetable peeler, remove a thin strip of skin from around the center of each potato. In large bowl, combine the oil, rosemary, mustard, sage, thyme, and pepper. Add the potatoes, and toss to combine.

Cut 4 (12"-long) pieces of foil. Divide the potato mixture evenly among the foil pieces. Tightly wrap the potatoes in the foil. Place the packets in the oven or on the grill. Cook, turning packets once, for 30–35 minutes in the oven or for 25–30 minutes on the grill, until the potatoes are tender.

Serves 4

NUTRITION AT A GLANCE

Per serving: 183 calories, 5 g protein,
30 g carbohydrates, 7 g fat, 1 g saturated fats,
0 mg sodium, 0 mg cholesterol, 4 g fiber

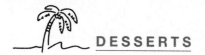

DESSERTS

Strawberries in Balsamic Vinegar

2 pints strawberries, stemmed and halved

2 packets sugar substitute

3 tablespoons balsamic vinegar

   Coarsely ground black pepper

   Mint sprigs (optional)

In a medium bowl, toss the strawberries, sugar substitute, and balsamic vinegar. Let stand at room temperature until ready to serve.

To serve, spoon into 4 dessert bowls. Grind a little black pepper over the tops. Garnish with mint sprigs, if using.

Serves 4

NUTRITION AT A GLANCE

Per serving: 59 calories, 1 g protein,
14 g carbohydrates, 1 g fat, 0 g saturated fats,
5 mg sodium, 0 mg cholesterol, 4 g fiber

Poached Pears

1 package (4-serving size) sugar-free raspberry or strawberry gelatin

2 cups boiling water

4 small pears, cored and peeled

In a saucepan large enough to hold all the pears, dissolve the gelatin in the boiling water. Add the pears and simmer gently, covered, for 8–10 minutes. Turn them a few times so that they will take on a uniform blush. Test with a cake tester or toothpick. When the pears offer no resistance when pierced, remove them with a slotted spoon. Do not overcook. Refrigerate when cool.

Pour the remaining gelatin into 4 small custard cups and chill until set.

Serves 4

NUTRITION AT A GLANCE

Per serving: 199 calories, 11 g protein,
25 g carbohydrates, 1 g fat, 0 g saturated fats,
549 mg sodium, 0 mg cholesterol, 4 g fiber

Ginger Pears

4 medium pears, peeled, halved, and cored

¼ cup fresh orange juice

½ cup finely crushed gingersnaps

2 tablespoons chopped walnuts

2 tablespoons margarine or butter

Preheat the oven to 350°F. Place the pear halves, cut side up, in a 12" x 7½" x 2" baking dish. Drizzle the orange juice over the pears. In a small bowl, combine the gingersnaps, walnuts, and the margarine or butter. Sprinkle over the pears. Bake for 20–25 minutes or until the fruit is tender.

Serves 8

NUTRITION AT A GLANCE

Per serving: 110 calories, 1 g protein, 16 g carbohydrates, 5 g fat, 1 g saturated fats, 55 mg sodium, 0 mg cholesterol, 2 g fiber

Individual Lime Cheesecakes

12 vanilla wafers

¾ cup fat-free cottage cheese

1 package (8 ounces) Neufchâtel cheese, softened

¼ cup + 2 tablespoons sugar

2 eggs

1 tablespoon grated lime rind

1 tablespoon fresh lime juice

1 teaspoon vanilla extract

¼ cup low-fat vanilla yogurt

2 medium kiwifruit, peeled, sliced, and halved

Preheat the oven to 350°F. Line 12 muffin pans with paper baking liners. Place 1 vanilla wafer in the bottom of each liner.

Process the cottage cheese in a blender or food processor until smooth. Combine the cottage cheese with the Neufchâtel in a medium bowl and beat at medium speed until creamy. Gradually add the sugar and mix well. Add the eggs, lime rind, lime juice, and vanilla. Beat until smooth. Spoon the cheese mixture evenly over the vanilla wafers. Bake at 350°F for 20 minutes or until the cheesecakes are almost set. (Do not overbake.) Let the cheesecakes cool completely on a wire rack. Remove from the pans and chill thoroughly.

Spread the vanilla yogurt evenly over the cheesecakes, and top each one with 3 kiwifruit slices.

Serves 12

NUTRITION AT A GLANCE

Per serving: 129 calories, 5 g protein,
13 g carbohydrates, 7 g fat, 3 g saturated fats,
161 mg sodium, 51 mg cholesterol, 1 g fiber

Chocolate Sponge Cake

7 egg whites

⅛ teaspoon cream of tartar

¾ cups sugar

3 egg yolks

1 teaspoon vanilla extract

1 cup sifted cake flour

3 tablespoons butter, melted and cooled to lukewarm

1½ ounces semisweet chocolate

2 tablespoons vegetable shortening

Preheat the oven to 350°F. In a large bowl, beat the egg whites with the cream of tartar until foamy. Beat in the sugar, 1 tablespoon at a time, until the meringue forms stiff, but not dry peaks. In another large bowl, stir together the egg yolks and vanilla. Fold in one-third of the meringue. Fold in the remaining meringue until no streaks of white remain. Sprinkle the cake flour over the top of the mixture and fold in. Very gently fold in the melted butter—do not overfold. Spoon the batter into a 10" tube pan, spreading evenly. Bake for 40–45 minutes or until a wooden pick inserted near the center comes out clean.

Invert the cake onto a large funnel or bottle. Let the cake hang until it is completely cooled, a minimum of 90 minutes. Run a knife around the inner and outer edges of the cake, turn out onto a rack, and cool completely with the crusty portion up.

Melt the chocolate together with the vegetable shortening in the top of a double boiler over hot, but not boiling water, stirring occasionally, until smooth. Cool slightly. Spoon the melted chocolate evenly over the top of the cake, letting the excess run down the sides.

Serves 10

NUTRITION AT A GLANCE

Per serving: 197 calories, 4 g protein, 26 g carbohydrates, 9 g fat, 4 g saturated fats, 76 mg sodium, 73 mg cholesterol, 0 g fiber

Chocolate-Stuffed Steamed Pears

  2 ripe Bartlett pears, washed

10 semisweet chocolate chips

Slice the top off of each pear, slightly above the widest part. Using a melon ball scoop or a small spoon, remove the cores from the bottom halves of the pears. Fill the hollowed pear bottoms with 5 chocolate chips each. Place the pear tops back on the bottoms.

    Stand each pear upright in an ovenproof custard cup. Set the cups in a medium saucepan and add 1" of water to the pan. Bring the water to a simmer over medium heat. Cover the pan and steam the pears for about 20 minutes, until translucent. Serve hot.

Serves 2

NUTRITION AT A GLANCE

Per serving: 179 calories, 2 g protein, 35 g carbohydrates, 5 g fat, 2 g saturated fats, 0 mg sodium, 1 mg cholesterol, 4 g fiber

Chocolate-Dipped Apricots

2　ounces bittersweet chocolate

24　dried apricots

1　tablespoon chopped pistachios

Microwave the chocolate in a microwaveable bowl on high for 2 minutes, stirring after 1 minute. Stir until completely melted. Dip the apricots halfway into the chocolate. Let the excess chocolate drip off. Place the apricots onto waxed paper. Sprinkle the pistachios over the chocolate-covered portions of the apricots. Place in the refrigerator until the chocolate is set.

Serves 8

NUTRITION AT A GLANCE

Per serving: 99 calories, 1 g protein,
17 g carbohydrates, 3 g fat, 2 g saturated fats,
1 mg sodium, 0 mg cholesterol, 2 g fiber

CREDITS

Recipe on page 138 used with permission of Roger Ruch, executive chef from 1220 at the Tides, Miami Beach.

Recipes on pages 144 and 278 used with permission of China Grill Management for China Grill, Miami Beach.

Recipes on pages 154 and 222 used with permission of China Grill Management for Tuscan Steak, Miami Beach.

Recipes on pages 174 and 226 used with permission of Andre Bienvenue, executive chef from Joe's Stone Crab, Miami Beach.

Recipe on page 206 used with permission of China Grill Management for Blue Door at Delano, Miami Beach.

Recipe on page 212 used with permission of Scott Fredel and J. D. Harris, executive chefs from Rumi Supper Club, Miami Beach.

Recipes on pages 234 and 284 used with permission of Michael D'Andrea, executive chef/owner from Macaluso's, Miami Beach.

Recipe for Armand Salad on page 164 is reprinted from *Eat at Joe's Cookbook,* and used with permission of Bay Books, © 2000.

INDEX

Underscored page references indicate boxed text and tables. **Boldface** references indicate photographs.

G

H

I

J

K

L

O

Oat bran, 42, 46

Oatmeal, 42, 46–47, 61, 62, 64

Oatmeal Pancake, 201

Obesity. *See also* Overweight

diabetes and, 75, 77–79

heart disease and, 79–80

Omelets

Easy Asparagus and Mushroom Omelet, 132

Western Egg White Omelet, 133

Onions

Oven-Roasted Vegetables, 168

Pan-Roasted Steak and Onions, 220

Roast Chicken with Sweet Garlic, Melted Onions, and Sour Orange, 268–69

Stewed Tomatoes and Onions, 172

Vegetable Quiche Cups to Go, 134

Orange juice

avoiding, 46

oranges vs., 47, 57

Orange roughy

Orange Roughy in Scallion and Ginger Sauce, 163

Oranges

vs. orange juice, 47, 57

Roast Chicken with Sweet Garlic, Melted Onions, and Sour Orange, 268–69

Oregano

Grilled Yellowfin Tuna with a White Bean and Oregano Salad, 222–23

Herb-Marinated Chicken, 217

Ornish, Dean, 22

Ornish plan, 9, 11, 22

Overweight. *See also* Obesity

from carbohydrates, 10

diabetes and, 78

health effects of, 7–8

P

Pancake

Oatmeal Pancake, 201

Parmesan cheese

Baked Tomatoes with Basil and Parmesan, 230

Pasta

glycemic index of, 72–73

whole wheat, in South Beach Diet, 11

Peanut butter and jelly sandwich, modifying, 49–50

Pears

Asian Pear Salad, 278–79

Chocolate-Stuffed Steamed Pears, 293

Ginger Pears, 290

Poached Pears, 289

Pecans

Endive and Pecan Salad, 261

Peppers, bell

Asian-Style Chicken Packets with Vegetables, 219

Beef, Pepper, and Mushroom Kabobs, 273

Oven-Roasted Vegetables, 168

Roasted Eggplant and Peppers, 169

Tuna, Cucumber, and Red Pepper Salad with Lemony Dill Dressing, 264

Vegetable Medley, 238

Vegetable Quiche Cups to Go, 134

Western Egg White Omelet, 133

Phase 1 of South Beach Diet

foods permitted in, 3–4, 126–27, 128

foods to avoid in, 127

guidelines for, 111

meal plans for, 112–25

starting, 25–30

Phase 2 of South Beach Diet

diet failure and, 101, 102

foods permitted in, 5, 183, 200

foods reintroduced to, 198

foods to avoid or eat rarely in, 199

guidelines for, 183

meal plans for, 184–97

Phase 3 of South Beach Diet

foods permitted in, 5

guidelines for, 243

meal plans for, 244–57

Phase 1 recipes, 128

breakfasts, 25–27

Artichokes Benedict, 135

Cheesy Frittata, 129

Easy Asparagus and Mushroom Omelet, 132

Light Spinach Frittata with Tomato Salsa, 130

Mock Hollandaise Sauce, 136

Smoked Salmon Frittata, 131

Q

R